病理学彩色图谱
COLOUR ATLAS OF PATHOLOGY

主 审 郑 杰
主 编 陈瑞芬 Zhang Deming（Canada）
副主编 董小黎 李 良 宫丽平 王蓬文
编 者（按拼音排序）

Zhang Deming（Victoria General Hospital，Winnipeg Canada）
陈瑞芬（首都医科大学）
董小黎（首都医科大学）
宫丽平（首都医科大学）
李 良（首都医科大学）
李海燕（首都医科大学）
廖 静（首都医科大学）
刘 瑜（首都医科大学）
任乐荣（首都医科大学）
时淑舫（首都医科大学附属友谊医院）
宋爱利（首都医科大学）
宋丽娜（首都医科大学）
孙 静（首都医科大学）
王 鹏（首都医科大学附属友谊医院）
王大业（首都医科大学）
王蓬文（首都医科大学）
王小平（首都医科大学）
杨 慧（首都医科大学）
张立洁（首都医科大学附属佑安医院）
郑 杰（北京大学医学部病理系）

科学出版社
北 京

内 容 简 介

本图谱精选428幅包括各种病变的肉眼和镜下图像，内容分为总论和各论两部分。总论图谱共151幅，其中包括细胞和组织的适应与损伤、损伤的修复、局部血液循环障碍、炎症和肿瘤的病变。各论图谱共277幅，其中包括心血管系统、呼吸系统、消化系统、淋巴造血系统、泌尿系统、生殖系统及传染病的常见病理变化及其特点。

本图谱可作为高等医学院校学生及其他各级医护院校学生的配套辅助教材，也可供医学专业工作者参考。

图书在版编目（CIP）数据

病理学彩色图谱/陈瑞芬等主编.—北京：科学出版社，2006.4
ISBN 978-7-03-016980-8

Ⅰ.病… Ⅱ.陈… Ⅲ.病理学－图谱 Ⅳ.R36-64
中国版本图书馆CIP数据核字（2006）第016199号

责任编辑：裴中惠／责任校对：宋玲玲
责任印制：赵 博／封面设计：黄 超

版权所有，违者必究。未经本社许可，数字图书馆不得使用

科学出版社 出版
北京东黄城根北街16号
邮政编码：100717
http://www.sciencep.com
北京建宏印刷有限公司印刷

科学出版社发行 各地新华书店经销
*
2006年4月第 一 版 开本：A5 890×1240
2024年7月第四次印刷 印张：5
字数：181 000
定价：49.80元

（如有印装质量问题，我社负责调换）

前 言

病理解剖学是通过形态学研究疾病的病因、发病机制、病理变化、结局和转归的医学基础学科，有很强的直观性。因此，无论在基础医学教学还是在临床医学诊断教学中，除了文字的参考书和教科书外，还需要与病理学教学图谱相配合，使病理改变图像化、理论问题形象化。特别是随着科学技术的不断发展，新的影像仪器和设备不断增加，图像分辨力不断提高，图像已日益成为诊断疾病不可缺少的手段。

本书选材主要依据普通高等医学院校教学大纲，紧密围绕五年制和七年制全国统编教材的主要内容，同时也兼顾高等职业院校的需要编写。通过图像帮助学生深入理解病理解剖的基本知识、基本理论，提高学生鉴别各种病理变化的基本技能。

图谱是在北京大学医学部病理系专家郑杰教授指导下，由首都医科大学病理解剖教研室具有丰富一线教学经验的老师与Victoria General Hospital，Winnipeg Canada的Dr. Zhang Deming，经过多年的努力与合作编写而成，在编写过程中注意在充分展示内容的同时，考虑到价格和学生的承受能力，因此从3000多幅肉眼和镜下标本的图片中精选出428幅编写了这本《病理学彩色图谱》。本图谱的特色为利用数字图像处理技术对图像进行加工，使病变的结构和特点更加突出；特别是用高分辨率的数码相机拍摄的肉眼标本，图像更清晰，颜色更逼真。图谱编写的过程中，着重在实用性的基础上力求内容先进，如在图谱中包含SARS的主要脏器的病理变化。本书资料来源于首都医科大学附属友谊医院、附属同仁医院、附属右安医院、Victoria General Hospital，Winnipeg Canada与首都医科大学病理解剖教研室。图谱得以顺利编写，与各位编者团结协作和精益求精的工作态度，特别是各医院病理科为我们提供了大量图像资料是分不开的，在此对他们表示一并致谢。科学出版社领导和编辑为图谱的出版给予了大力的支持，在此表示深深的感谢。

在图谱的编写过程中，虽然主编与编者付出了很大的努力，力求做到完美，但由于我们的学术水平和实践经验有限，难免会出现一些缺点和错误，希望各位教师和学生提出宝贵意见，恳切希望给予批评和指正，以便今后进一步修订和完善。

编 者

2006年1月19日

目 录

第 1 篇 病理学总论
GENERAL PATHOLOGY

图 1　肝细胞萎缩 Atrophy of liver ··2
图 2　肾压迫性萎缩 Pressure atrophy of kidney ···························2
图 3　心脏褐色萎缩 Brown atrophy of heart ·······························2
图 4　子宫肥大 Hypertrophy of uterus ·······································3
图 5　鼻息肉腺体增生 Gland hyperplasia of polyp，nose ···············3
图 6　胃黏膜肠上皮化生 Intestine metaplasia of stomach ···············3
图 7　肝细胞水肿 Cellular swelling of hepatocytes ·······················4
图 8　心肌细胞水肿 Cellular swelling of myocytes ·······················4
图 9　肝脂肪变性 Fatty change of liver ····································4
图 10　肝细胞脂肪变 Fatty change of liver ································5
图 11　肝细胞玻璃样变 Hyaline degeneration of liver ···················5
图 12　浆细胞 Rusell 小体 Rusell body of plasma cell ···················5
图 13　纤维结缔组织玻璃样变 Hyaline degeneration of connective tissues ···6
图 14　脾中央动脉玻璃样变 Hyaline degeneration of spleen central arteriole ···6
图 15　心肌淀粉样变 Amyloidosis of heart ·································6
图 16　心肌淀粉样变 Amyloidosis of heart ·································7
图 17　胎盘钙化 Calcification of placenta ·································7
图 18　胰腺凝固性坏死 Coagulative necrosis of pancreas ···············7
图 19　心肌凝固性坏死 Coagulative necrosis of heart ···················8
图 20　肾凝固性坏死 Coagulative necrosis of kidney ····················8
图 21　胰腺液化性坏死 Liquefactive necrosis of pancreas ···············8
图 22　心肌脓肿（液化性坏死） Abscess of heart（liquefactive necrosis） ···9
图 23　动脉壁纤维素样坏死 Fibrinoid necrosis of artery ················9
图 24　阑尾湿性坏疽 Moist gangrene of appendix ·······················9
图 25　淋巴结核干酪样坏死 Caseous necrosis of lymph node ········10
图 26　淋巴结核干酪样坏死 Caseous necrosis of lymph node ········10
图 27　肺结核空洞形成 Tubercular cavity of lung ······················10
图 28　肝细胞凋亡 Apoptosis of liver ·····································11
图 29　分泌期腺体的凋亡 Apoptosis of secretory gland ···············11
图 30　肝细胞凋亡 Apoptosis of hepatocytes ····························11
图 31　巨噬细胞吞噬凋亡小体 Apoptosis body engulfed by macrophage ···12

图 32	肉芽组织 Granulation tissue	12
图 33	瘢痕组织 Scar tissue	12
图 34	I 期愈合 Healing by first intention	13
图 35	脾淤血 Spleen congestion	13
图 36	肺淤血 Lung congestion	13
图 37	肺淤血 Lung congestion	14
图 38	慢性肺淤血（心衰细胞）Chronic lung congestion（heart failure cells）	14
图 39	急性肝淤血 Acute liver congestion	14
图 40	慢性肝淤血 Chronic liver congestion	15
图 41	槟榔肝 Nutmeg liver	15
图 42	血栓形成 – 血小板黏附 Thrombosis-platelets adhesion	15
图 43	血栓形成 – 血小板伪足 Thrombosis-pseudopod of platelet	16
图 44	血小板性血栓 Platelet thrombus	16
图 45	白色血栓 Pale thrombus	16
图 46	白色血栓（PTAH 染色，同图 45）Pale thrombus（PTAH staining, same as above figure）	17
图 47	胰腺小叶间动脉混合血栓 Mixed thrombus of artery in pancreas	17
图 48	心脏室壁瘤伴附壁血栓形成 Ventricular aneurysm with mural thrombosis	17
图 49	动脉内混合血栓 Mixed thrombus of artery	18
图 50	脑膜血管内血栓 Thrombus of meningeal blood vessel	18
图 51	动脉内混合血栓 Mixed thrombus of artery	18
图 52	DIC 肾小球毛细血管内微血栓形成 Microthrombosis of glomerulus during DIC	19
图 53	肾小球内微血栓形成（PTAH 染色）Microthrombosis of glomerulus（PTAH staining）	19
图 54	血栓机化再通 Thrombus organization and recanalization	19
图 55	血栓再通 Thrombus recanalization	20
图 56	血栓钙化 Thrombus calcification	20
图 57	肺动脉血栓栓塞 Pulmonary thromboembolism	20
图 58	肺血管脂肪栓塞 Pulmonary fat embolism	21
图 59	肾血管脂肪栓塞（胆固醇栓子）Renal fat embolism（cholesterin embolus）	21
图 60	脾贫血性梗死 Anemic infarct of spleen	21
图 61	心肌梗死 Myocardial infarction	22
图 62	肺出血性梗死 Hemorrhagic infarct of lung	22
图 63	肠出血性梗死 Hemorrhagic infarct of intestine	22
图 64	肠出血性梗死 Hemorrhagic infarct of intestine	22
图 65	中性粒细胞 Neutrophil	23
图 66	浆细胞 Plasma cell	23
图 67	淋巴细胞 Lymphocyte	23

iii

图 68　嗜酸粒细胞 Eosinophil ······24
图 69　白细胞附壁 Leukocytic adhesion ······24
图 70　白细胞的游出 Leukocytic emigration ······24
图 71　红细胞的漏出 Red cells leak ······25
图 72　白细胞的吞噬作用 Leukocytic phagocytosis ······25
图 73　气管纤维素性炎 Fibrinous inflammation of trachea ······25
图 74　肠纤维素性炎 Fibrinous inflammation of intestine ······25
图 75　肠纤维素性炎 Fibrinous inflammation of intestine ······26
图 76　纤维素性心外膜炎 Fibrinous pericarditis ······26
图 77　胸膜纤维素性炎 Fibrinous inflammation of pleura ······26
图 78　肺纤维素性炎 Fibrinous inflammation of lung ······26
图 79　化脓性腹膜炎 Suppurative peritonitis ······27
图 80　化脓性脑膜炎 Suppurative meningitis ······27
图 81　化脓性脑膜炎 Suppurative meningitis ······27
图 82　急性蜂窝织炎性阑尾炎 Acute phlegmonous appendicitis ······28
图 83　急性蜂窝织炎性阑尾炎 Acute phlegmonous appendicitis ······28
图 84　急性蜂窝织炎性阑尾炎 Acute phlegmonous appendicitis ······28
图 85　毛囊炎 Folliculitis ······29
图 86　脑脓肿 Cerebral abscess ······29
图 87　脓肿 Abscess ······29
图 88　脓肿 Abscess ······30
图 89　慢性胃炎 Chronic gastritis ······30
图 90　慢性子宫内膜炎 Chronic endometritis ······30
图 91　慢性胆囊炎 Chronic cholecystitis ······31
图 92　慢性胆囊炎 Chronic cholecystitis ······31
图 93　肠息肉 Polyp of intestine ······31
图 94　肠息肉 Polyp of intestine ······32
图 95　鼻炎性息肉 Inflammatory polyp, nose ······32
图 96　异物肉芽肿 Foreign body granuloma ······32
图 97　结核结节 Tubercle ······33
图 98　皮肤乳头状瘤 Papilloma of skin ······33
图 99　皮肤乳头状瘤 Papilloma of skin ······33
图 100　卵巢浆液性囊腺瘤 Serous cystadenoma of ovary ······34
图 101　卵巢浆液性囊腺瘤 Serous cystadenoma of ovary ······34
图 102　卵巢黏液性囊腺瘤 Mucinous cystadenoma of ovary ······34
图 103　卵巢黏液性囊腺瘤 Mucinous cystadenoma of ovary ······35
图 104　甲状旁腺腺瘤 Parathyroid adenoma ······35
图 105　子宫内膜非典型性增生 Endometrial atypical hyperplasia ······35

图 106　胰腺原位癌 Carcinoma in situ of pancreas··36
图 107　皮肤鳞癌 Squamous carcinoma of skin··36
图 108　高分化鳞癌 Well differentiated squamous carcinoma··································36
图 109　直肠肛门鳞癌 Squamous carcinoma of rectum··37
图 110　结肠癌 Carcinoma of colon··37
图 111　结肠腺癌 Adenocarcinoma of colon···37
图 112　盲肠腺癌 Adenocarcinoma of cecum···38
图 113　卵巢浆液性囊腺癌 Serous cystadenocarcinoma of ovary··························38
图 114　高分化子宫内膜样腺癌 Well differentiated endomertrioid adenocarcinoma·····38
图 115　低分化子宫内膜样腺癌 Poorly differentiated endomertrioid adenocarcinoma···39
图 116　子宫内膜样腺癌 Endomertrioid adenocarcinoma······································39
图 117　子宫内膜浆液性乳头状癌 Endometrial serous papillary carcinoma········39
图 118　弥漫型胃腺癌 Diffuse adenocarcinoma of stomach···································40
图 119　胃印戒细胞癌 Signet-ring cell carcinoma of stomach································40
图 120　胃印戒细胞癌 Signet-ring cell carcinoma of stomach································40
图 121　胰腺导管腺癌 Ductal adenocarcinoma of pancreas··································41
图 122　低分化胰腺癌 Poorly differentiated carcinoma of pancreas····················41
图 123　甲状腺滤泡状腺癌（低倍镜）Thyroid follicular adenocarcinoma··········41
图 124　甲状腺滤泡状腺癌（高倍镜）Thyroid follicular adenocarcinoma··········42
图 125　甲状腺乳头状癌 Thyroid papillary carcinoma··42
图 126　肝癌腹膜种植转移 Liver carcinoma seeding to peritoneum······················42
图 127　纤维瘤 Fibroma··43
图 128　纤维瘤 Fibroma··43
图 129　乳腺纤维腺瘤 Fibroadenama of breast···43
图 130　脂肪瘤 Lipoma···44
图 131　脂肪瘤 Lipoma···44
图 132　脂肪瘤 Lipoma···44
图 133　子宫平滑肌瘤 Leiomyoma of uterus··45
图 134　子宫平滑肌瘤 Leiomyoma of uterus··45
图 135　骨肉瘤 Osteosarcoma···45
图 136　纤维肉瘤 Fibrosarcoma··46
图 137　横纹肌肉瘤 Rhabdomyosarcoma···46
图 138　平滑肌肉瘤（低倍镜）Leiomyosarcoma··46
图 139　平滑肌肉瘤（高倍镜）Leiomyosarcoma··47
图 140　皮肤血管肉瘤 Hemangiosarcoma of skin··47
图 141　脂肪肉瘤 Liposarcoma···47
图 142　脂肪肉瘤 Liposarcoma···48
图 143　混合痣（低倍镜）Junctional nevus··48

图 144　混合痣（高倍镜）Junctional nevus ··48
图 145　背部黑色素瘤 Melanoma of back ···49
图 146　背部黑色素瘤 Melanoma of back ···49
图 147　前臂痣恶变的黑色素瘤 Melanoma from nevus of forearm ···············49
图 148　卵巢囊性成熟性畸胎瘤 Mature cystic teratoma of ovary ·················50
图 149　卵巢囊性成熟性畸胎瘤 Mature cystic teratoma of ovary ·················50
图 150　卵巢实性成熟性畸胎瘤 Mature solid teratoma of ovary ···················50
图 151　卵巢成熟性畸胎瘤 Mature teratoma of ovary ·································50

第 2 篇　病理学各论
SYSTEMIC PATHOLOGY

图 152　纤维斑块 Fibrous plaque ··52
图 153　粥样斑块 Atheromatous plaque ··52
图 154　脂纹 Fatty streak ··53
图 155　粥样斑块 Atheromatous plaque ··53
图 156　粥样斑块 Atheromatous plaque ··53
图 157　斑块内出血 Hemorrhage in atheromatous plaque ·····························54
图 158　斑块破裂 Cracking of atheromatous plaque ····································54
图 159　斑块钙化 Calcification of atheromatous plaque ································54
图 160　脑动脉粥样硬化 Cerebral artery atherosclerosis ······························55
图 161　冠状动脉粥样硬化 Coronary atherosclerosis ···································55
图 162　冠状动脉粥样硬化 Coronary atherosclerosis ···································55
图 163　陈旧性心肌梗死 Stale myocardial infarction ···································56
图 164　心肌梗死 Myocardial infarction ··56
图 165　心肌梗死 Myocardial infarction ··56
图 166　心脏破裂 Rupture of heart ···57
图 167　心包填塞 Tamponade in pericardium ···57
图 168　高血压心脏病合并主动脉粥样硬化 Hypertensive heart disease with aorta atherosclerosis ···57
图 169　原发性颗粒性固缩肾 Primary granular atrophy of kidney ··················58
图 170　原发性颗粒性固缩肾 Primary granular atrophy of kidney ··················58
图 171　原发性颗粒性固缩肾 Primary granular atrophy of kidney ··················58
图 172　原发性颗粒性固缩肾 Primary granular atrophy of kidney ··················59
图 173　原发性颗粒性固缩肾 Primary granular atrophy of kidney ··················59
图 174　原发性颗粒性固缩肾 Primary granular atrophy of kidney ··················59
图 175　脑出血 Haemorrhage in cerebra ···60
图 176　脑出血 Haemorrhage in cerebra ···60

图 177　风湿小结 Aschoff body ···60
图 178　风湿细胞 Aschoff cell ··61
图 179　风湿性心内膜炎 Rheumatic endocarditis ··61
图 180　风湿性心外膜炎 Rheumatic pericarditis ··61
图 181　急性感染性心内膜炎 Acute infective endocarditis ······································62
图 182　亚急性感染性心内膜炎 Subacute infective endocarditis ·····························62
图 183　慢性瓣膜病 Chronic valvular vitium of heart ··62
图 184　慢性瓣膜病 Chronic valvular vitium of heart ··63
图 185　大叶性肺炎（灰色肝样变期）Lobar pneumonia（stage of gray hepatization） ······63
图 186　大叶性肺炎（灰色肝样变早期）Lobar pneumonia
　　　　（early stage of gray hepatization） ···63
图 187　大叶性肺炎（灰色肝样变早期）Lobar pneumonia（stage of gray hepatization） ···64
图 188　小叶性肺炎 Lobular pneumonia ··64
图 189　小叶性肺炎 Lobular pneumonia ··64
图 190　病毒性肺炎（病毒包涵体）Viral pneumonia（viral inclusion bodies） ··········65
图 191　严重急性呼吸综合征（SARS）Severe acute respiratory syndrome ··············65
图 192　严重急性呼吸综合征（SARS）Severe acute respiratory syndrome ··············65
图 193　严重急性呼吸综合征（SARS）Severe acute respiratory syndrome ··············66
图 194　严重急性呼吸综合征（SARS）Severe acute respiratory syndrome ··············66
图 195　严重急性呼吸综合征（SARS）Severe acute respiratory syndrome ··············66
图 196　严重急性呼吸综合征（SARS）（肺门淋巴结）Severe acute respiratory
　　　　syndrome（lymph node at hilum of lung） ··67
图 197　严重急性呼吸综合征（SARS）伴曲菌感染 Severe acute respiratory
　　　　syndrome with aspergillus infection ···67
图 198　支气管哮喘 Bronchial asthma ··67
图 199　支气管扩张症 Bronchiectasis ··68
图 200　肺气肿 Pulmonary emphysema ···68
图 201　肺气肿 Pulmonary emphysema ···68
图 202　间质性肺气肿 Interstitial emphysema ···69
图 203　硅肺 Silicosis ··69
图 204　肺心病 Cor pulmonale ··69
图 205　新生儿呼吸窘迫综合征（NRDS）Neonatal respiratory distress syndrome ······70
图 206　颈淋巴结转移性鼻咽癌（非角化型鳞癌）Neck lymph node with metastatic
　　　　nasopharyngeal carcinoma（nonkeratinizing squamous cell carcinoma） ···········70
图 207　颈淋巴结转移性鼻咽癌（非角化型鳞癌）Neck lymph node with metastatic
　　　　nasopharyngeal carcinoma（nonkeratinizing squamous cell carcinoma） ···········70
图 208　中央型肺癌 Carcinoma of lung, central type ···71
图 209　周围型肺癌 Carcinoma of lung, peripheral type ··71

图 210	肺鳞癌 Squamous cell carcinoma of lung	71
图 211	肺腺癌（混合细胞型）Adenocarcinoma of lung (mixed cell subtype)	72
图 212	肺腺癌（杯状细胞型）Adenocarcinoma of lung (goblet cell subtype)	72
图 213	肺腺癌（细支气管肺泡癌）Adenocarcinoma of lung (bronchioloalveolar carcinoma)	72
图 214	肺小细胞癌 Small cell carcinoma of lung	73
图 215	肺大细胞癌 Large cell carcinoma of lung	73
图 216	肺类癌 Carcinoid of lung	73
图 217	肺类癌 Carcinoid of lung	74
图 218	胸膜间皮瘤 Pleural mesothelioma	74
图 219	胸膜间皮瘤 Pleural mesothelioma	74
图 220	反流性食管炎 Regurgitant esophagitis	75
图 221	白色念珠菌食管炎 Candida albicans esophagitis	75
图 222	幽门螺杆菌性胃炎 H. pylori gastritis	75
图 223	幽门螺杆菌性胃炎（Giemsa 染色）H. pylori gastritis	76
图 224	慢性萎缩性胃炎 Chronic atrophic gastritis	76
图 225	胃肠上皮化生 Intestinal metaplasia of stomach	76
图 226	胃溃疡 Gastric ulcer	77
图 227	急性化脓性阑尾炎 Acute suppurative appendicitis	77
图 228	急性化脓性阑尾炎 Acute suppurative appendicitis	77
图 229	急性化脓性阑尾炎 Acute suppurative appendicitis	78
图 230	急性坏疽性阑尾炎 Acute gangrenous appendicitis	78
图 231	急性坏疽性阑尾炎 Acute gangrenous appendicitis	78
图 232	慢性阑尾炎 Chronic appendicitis	79
图 233	Crohn 病 Crohn's disease	79
图 234	慢性溃疡性结肠炎 Chronic ulcerative colitis	79
图 235	Meckel 憩室 Meckel's diverticulum	80
图 236	急性病毒性肝炎 Acute viral hepatitis	80
图 237	慢性肝炎,桥接坏死 Chronic hepatitis, bridging necrosis	80
图 238	酒精性肝炎 Alcoholic hepatitis	81
图 239	门脉性肝硬化 Portal cirrhosis	81
图 240	门脉性肝硬化 Portal cirrhosis	81
图 241	食管下段静脉曲张 Esophageal varices	82
图 242	原发性胆汁性肝硬化 Primary biliary cirrhosis	82
图 243	肝血色病 Liver hemochromatosis	82
图 244	急性胆囊炎 Acute cholecystitis	83
图 245	慢性胆囊炎 Chronic cholecystitis	83
图 246	食管癌 Carcinoma of esophagus	83

图 247	食管鳞癌 Squamous cell carcinoma of esophagus	84
图 248	溃疡型胃癌 Ulcerative type of gastric carcinoma	84
图 249	胃腺癌 Adenocarcinoma of stomach	84
图 250	弥漫性浸润型胃癌 Diffuse invasive type of gastric carcinoma	85
图 251	弥漫性浸润型胃癌 Diffuse invasive type of gastric carcinoma	85
图 252	胃腺癌 Adenocarcinoma of stomach	85
图 253	胃黏液癌（低倍镜）Mucinous carcinoma of stomach	86
图 254	胃黏液癌（高倍镜）Mucinous carcinoma of stomach	86
图 255	胃印戒细胞癌 Signet-ring cell carcinoma of stomach	86
图 256	胃小细胞癌（低倍镜）Small cell carcinoma of stomach	87
图 257	胃小细胞癌（高倍镜）Small cell carcinoma of stomach	87
图 258	胃癌肝转移 Metastatic gastric carcinoma in liver	87
图 259	胃平滑肌瘤（低倍镜）Leiomyoma of stomach	88
图 260	胃平滑肌瘤（高倍镜）Leiomyoma of stomach	88
图 261	胃底腺息肉 Fundic gland polyp	88
图 262	胃增生性息肉 Hyperplastic polyp of stomach	89
图 263	溃疡型直肠癌 Ulcerative type of rectal carcinoma	89
图 264	隆起型肠癌 Massive type of intestinal carcinoma	89
图 265	结肠腺癌（低倍镜）Adenocarcinoma of colon	90
图 266	结肠腺癌（高倍镜）Adenocarcinoma of colon	90
图 267	结肠腺癌凋亡 Apoptosis of colon adenocarcinoma cells	90
图 268	结肠腺癌淋巴结转移 Metastatic colon adenocarcinoma in lymph node	91
图 269	小肠类癌 Carcinoid tumor of small bowel	91
图 270	结肠管状腺瘤 Tubular adenoma of colon	91
图 271	结肠绒毛状腺瘤 Villus adenoma of colon	92
图 272	直肠平滑肌瘤 Leiomyoma of rectum	92
图 273	结肠 Peutz-Jephers 息肉 Peutz-Jephers polyp of colon	92
图 274	阑尾黏液囊腺瘤 Mucinous cystadenoma of appendix	93
图 275	阑尾黏液囊腺瘤 Mucinous cystadenoma of appendix	93
图 276	肝细胞癌 Hepatocellular carcinoma	93
图 277	胆囊腺癌 Adenocarcinoma of gallbladder	94
图 278	胰头癌 Carcinoma of head of pancreas	94
图 279	胰腺导管腺癌 Ductal adenocarcinoma of pancreas	94
图 280	弥漫性大 B 细胞淋巴瘤（远端回肠）Diffuse large-B cell lymphoma（distal ileum）	95
图 281	弥漫性大 B 细胞淋巴瘤（远端回肠）Diffuse large-B cell lymphoma（distal ileum）	95
图 282	弥漫性大 B 细胞淋巴瘤 Diffuse large-B cell lymphoma	95

图 283	弥漫性大 B 细胞淋巴瘤 Diffuse large-B cell lymphoma	96
图 284	弥漫性大 B 细胞淋巴瘤（腋下淋巴结） Diffuse large-B cell lymphoma（axillary lymph node）	96
图 285	滤泡性淋巴瘤（颈部淋巴结）Follicular lymphoma (cervical lymph node)	96
图 286	滤泡性淋巴瘤（1 级）Follicular lymphoma (grade 1)	97
图 287	滤泡性淋巴瘤（2 级）Follicular lymphoma (grade 2)	97
图 288	黏膜相关淋巴组织（MALT）淋巴瘤 Mucosa-associated lymphoid tissue lymphoma	97
图 289	黏膜相关淋巴组织（MALT）淋巴瘤 Mucosa-associated lymphoid tissue lymphoma	98
图 290	黏膜相关淋巴组织（MALT）淋巴瘤 Mucosa-associated lymphoid tissue lymphoma	98
图 291	慢性淋巴细胞性白血病/小细胞淋巴瘤病 Chronic lymphocytic leukaemia/small lymphocytic lymphoma	98
图 292	慢性淋巴细胞性白血病/小细胞淋巴瘤病 Chronic lymphocytic leukaemia/small lymphocytic lymphoma	99
图 293	慢性淋巴细胞性白血病/小细胞淋巴瘤病 Chronic lymphocytic leukaemia/small lymphocytic lymphoma	99
图 294	套细胞淋巴瘤（骨）Mantle cell lymphoma (bone)	99
图 295	淋巴浆细胞性淋巴瘤 Lymphoplasmacytic lymphoma	100
图 296	多发性骨髓瘤 Multiple myeloma	100
图 297	多发性骨髓瘤 Multiple myeloma	100
图 298	Burkitt 样淋巴瘤 Burkitt-like lymphoma	101
图 299	Burkitt 样淋巴瘤 Burkitt-like lymphoma	101
图 300	外周 T 细胞淋巴瘤（非特异性）Peripheral T-cell lymphoma (unspecified)	101
图 301	外周 T 细胞淋巴瘤（非特异性）Peripheral T-cell lymphoma (unspecified)	102
图 302	NK/T 细胞淋巴瘤 NK/T-cell lymphoma	102
图 303	T 淋巴母细胞性淋巴瘤 T-lymphoblastic lymphoma	102
图 304	T 淋巴母细胞性淋巴瘤 T-lymphoblastic lymphoma	103
图 305	间变性大细胞淋巴瘤 Anaplastic large cell lymphoma	103
图 306	血管免疫母细胞性 T 细胞淋巴瘤 Angioimmunoblastic T-cell lymphoma	103
图 307	结节性淋巴细胞为主型霍奇金淋巴瘤 Nodular lymphocyte predominant Hodgkin lymphoma	104
图 308	结节性淋巴细胞为主型霍奇金淋巴瘤 Nodular lymphocyte predominant Hodgkin lymphoma	104
图 309	结节性淋巴细胞为主型霍奇金淋巴瘤 Nodular lymphocyte predominant Hodgkin lymphoma	104

图 310	结节性淋巴细胞为主型霍奇金淋巴瘤	
	Nodular lymphocyte predominant Hodgkin lymphoma	105
图 311	经典型霍奇金淋巴瘤（结节硬化亚型）	
	Classical Hodgkin lymphoma（nodular sclerosis subtype）	105
图 312	经典型霍奇金淋巴瘤（结节硬化亚型）	
	Classical Hodgkin lymphoma（nodular sclerosis subtype）	105
图 313	经典型霍奇金淋巴瘤（混合细胞亚型）	
	Classical Hodgkin lymphoma（mixed cellularity subtype）	106
图 314	正常肾小球 Normal glomerulus	106
图 315	正常肾小球（电镜）Ultrastructure of normal glomerulus	106
图 316	免疫复合物沉积（免疫荧光）Deposition of immune complexes	
	（immunofluorescence）	107
图 317	急性弥漫性增生性肾小球肾炎 Acute diffuse proliferative	
	glomerulonephritis	107
图 318	急性弥漫性增生性肾小球肾炎（电镜）	
	Ultrastructure of acute diffuse proliferative glomerulonephritis	107
图 319	新月体性肾小球肾炎 Crescentic glomerulonephritis，CrGN	108
图 320	新月体性肾小球肾炎（环形小体）	
	Crescentic glomerulonephritis，CrGN	108
图 321	轻微病变性肾小球肾炎（电镜）	
	Ultrastructure of minimal change glomerulonephritis	108
图 322	继发性颗粒性固缩肾 Secondary granular atrophy of kidney	109
图 323	慢性肾小球肾炎 Chronic glomerulonephritis	109
图 324	慢性肾小球肾炎 Chronic glomerulonephritis	109
图 325	慢性肾小球肾炎 Chronic glomerulonephritis	110
图 326	慢性肾盂肾炎 Chronic pyelonephritis	110
图 327	慢性肾盂肾炎 Chronic pyelonephritis	110
图 328	慢性肾盂肾炎 Chronic pyelonephritis	111
图 329	慢性肾盂肾炎急性发作 Acute paroxysm of chronic pyelonephritis	111
图 330	慢性肾盂肾炎急性发作 Acute paroxysm of chronic pyelonephritis	111
图 331	肾细胞癌 Renal cell carcinoma	112
图 332	肾细胞癌 Renal cell carcinoma	112
图 333	肾透明细胞癌 Clear cell renal carcinoma	112
图 334	肾嫌色细胞癌 Chromophobe renal carcinoma	113
图 335	肾盂移行细胞癌 Transitional cell carcinoma of renal pelvis	113
图 336	肾盂移行细胞癌 Transitional cell carcinoma of renal pelvis	113
图 337	输尿管移行细胞癌 Transitional cell carcinoma of ureter	114
图 338	膀胱癌 Carcinoma of bladder	114

图 339	膀胱癌 Carcinoma of bladder	114
图 340	膀胱移行细胞原位癌 Transitional cell carcinoma in situ of bladder	115
图 341	膀胱乳头状移行上皮细胞癌 Papillary transitional cell carcinoma of bladder	115
图 342	膀胱乳头状移行上皮细胞癌 Papillary transitional cell carcinoma of bladder	115
图 343	膀胱浸润性移行细胞癌 Invasive transitional cell carcinoma of bladder	116
图 344	膀胱炎伴鳞状上皮化生 Cystitis with squamous metaplasia	116
图 345	膀胱炎伴鳞状上皮化生 Cystitis with squamous metaplasia	116
图 346	膀胱鳞癌原位癌 Squamous cell carcinoma in situ of bladder	117
图 347	膀胱高分化鳞癌 Well differentiated squamous cell carcinoma of bladder	117
图 348	多囊肾 Polycystic kidney	117
图 349	多囊肾 Polycystic kidney	118
图 350	慢性宫颈炎 Chronic cervicitis	118
图 351	子宫颈囊肿 Nabothian cyst	118
图 352	子宫颈上皮内瘤变Ⅰ级 Cervical intraepithelial neoplasia, CIN Ⅰ	119
图 353	子宫颈上皮内瘤变Ⅱ级 Cervical intraepithelial neoplasia, CIN Ⅱ	119
图 354	子宫颈上皮内瘤变Ⅲ级 Cervical intraepithelial neoplasia, CIN Ⅲ	119
图 355	子宫颈原位癌累及腺体 Carcinoma in situ of cervix and involved gland	120
图 356	子宫颈癌（内生浸润型）Carcinoma of cervix (invasive type)	120
图 357	子宫颈鳞状细胞癌（低分化）Squamous cell carcinoma of cervix (poorly differentiated)	120
图 358	子宫颈腺癌 Adenocarcinoma of cervix	121
图 359	子宫腺肌病 Adenomyosis of uterus	121
图 360	子宫腺肌病 Adenomyosis of uterus	121
图 361	子宫内膜单纯性增生 Simple hyperplasia of endometrium	122
图 362	子宫内膜复杂性增生 Complex hyperplasia of endometrium	122
图 363	子宫内膜非典型增生 Atypical hyperplasia of endometrium	122
图 364	子宫内膜癌（弥漫型）Adenocarcinoma of endometrium (diffuse type)	123
图 365	子宫内膜腺癌（高分化）Adenocarcinoma of endometrium (well differentiated)	123
图 366	子宫内膜腺癌（中分化）Adenocarcinoma of endometrium (moderate differentiated)	123
图 367	子宫内膜腺癌（低分化）Adenocarcinoma of endometrium (poorly differentiated)	124
图 368	子宫平滑肌瘤 Leiomyoma of uterus	124
图 369	子宫平滑肌瘤 Leiomyoma of uterus	124

图 370	子宫平滑肌瘤 Leiomyoma of uterus	125
图 371	葡萄胎（完全性）Hydatidiform mole（complete）	125
图 372	葡萄胎（完全性）Hydatidiform mole（complete）	125
图 373	葡萄胎（部分性）Hydatidiform mole（partial）	126
图 374	葡萄胎（部分性）Hydatidiform mole（partial）	126
图 375	侵蚀性葡萄胎 Invasive mole	126
图 376	子宫绒毛膜癌 Choriocarcinoma	127
图 377	子宫绒毛膜癌 Choriocarcinoma	127
图 378	子宫绒毛膜癌 Choriocarcinoma	127
图 379	子宫绒癌肝转移 Choriocarcinoma metastasis to liver	128
图 380	卵巢交界性浆液性乳头状囊腺瘤 Borderline serous papillary cystadenoma of ovary	128
图 381	卵巢浆液性乳头状囊腺癌 Serous papillary cystadenocarcinoma of ovary	128
图 382	卵巢成熟畸胎瘤 Mature teratoma of ovary	129
图 383	乳腺增生性纤维囊性变 Hyperplasia fibrocystic change of breast	129
图 384	乳腺硬化性腺病 Sclerosing adenosis of breast	129
图 385	乳腺纤维腺瘤 Fibroadenoma of breast	130
图 386	乳腺粉刺癌 Comedocarcinoma of breast	130
图 387	乳腺导管内原位癌 Intraductal carcinoma in situ of breast	130
图 388	乳腺导管内原位癌 Intraductal carcinoma in situ of breast	131
图 389	乳腺小叶原位癌 Lobular carcinoma in situ of breast	131
图 390	乳腺 Paget 病 Paget's disease of breast	131
图 391	乳腺癌 Carcinoma of breast	132
图 392	乳腺癌 Carcinoma of breast	132
图 393	乳腺浸润性导管癌 Invasive ductal carcinoma of breast	132
图 394	乳腺浸润性导管癌（硬癌）Invasive ductal carcinoma of breast（scirrhous carcinoma）	133
图 395	乳腺浸润性小叶癌 Invasive lobular carcinoma of breast	133
图 396	乳腺髓样癌 Medullary carcinoma of breast	133
图 397	乳腺黏液癌 Mucinous carcinoma of breast	134
图 398	原发进行性肺结核 Primary progressive pulmonary tuberculosis	134
图 399	干酪性肺炎 Caseous pneumonia	134
图 400	肺结核球 Pulmonary tuberculoma	135
图 401	肺结核球 Pulmonary tuberculoma	135
图 402	慢性纤维空洞型肺结核 Chronic fibro-cavitative pulmonary tuberculosis	135
图 403	粟粒性肺结核 Miliary tuberculosis of lung	136
图 404	脾粟粒性结核 Miliary tuberculosis of spleen	136
图 405	肺结核结节 Tubercle of lung	136

图 406　结核结节 Tubercle ···137
图 407　淋巴结结核 Tuberculosis of lymph nodes ·······································137
图 408　淋巴结结核 Tuberculosis of lymph nodes ·······································137
图 409　肾结核 Tuberculosis of kidney ···138
图 410　结核菌抗酸染色 Anti-acid stain of tubercle bacillus ························138
图 411　骨结核 Tuberculosis of bone ··138
图 412　肺结核钙化灶 Calcification of pulmonary tuberculosis ····················139
图 413　肠伤寒髓样肿胀期 Typhoid fever of intestine, stage of medullary swelling ······139
图 414　伤寒小结 Typhoid nodule ··139
图 415　假膜性肠炎 Pseudomembrane enteritis ··140
图 416　阿米巴痢疾的结肠 Amoebiasis of colon ··140
图 417　扁桃体放线菌 Tonsil actinomycete ···140
图 418　曲菌感染（PAS 染色）Aspergillus infection (PAS stain) ·················141
图 419　血吸虫虫卵 Eggs of schitosoma ···141
图 420　血吸虫病慢性虫卵结节 Chronic egg tubercle of schistosomiasis ·······141
图 421　细粒棘球蚴病 Echinococosis ··142
图 422　乙脑时嗜神经细胞象 Epidemic encephalitis B, engulfing nerve cells ··········142
图 423　乙脑时淋巴血管套 Epidemic encephalitis B, lymphocytes infiltrating around vessel ··142
图 424　乙脑时胶质细胞结节 Epidemic encephalitis B, nodule of glial cells ·······143
图 425　流行性脑脊髓膜炎 Epidemic cerebrospinal meningitis ·····················143
图 426　尖锐湿疣 Condyloma acuminatum ···143
图 427　尖锐湿疣 Condyloma acuminatum ···144
图 428　卡波西肉瘤 Kaposi's sarcoma ··144

病理学总论
GENERAL PATHOLOGY

第 1 篇

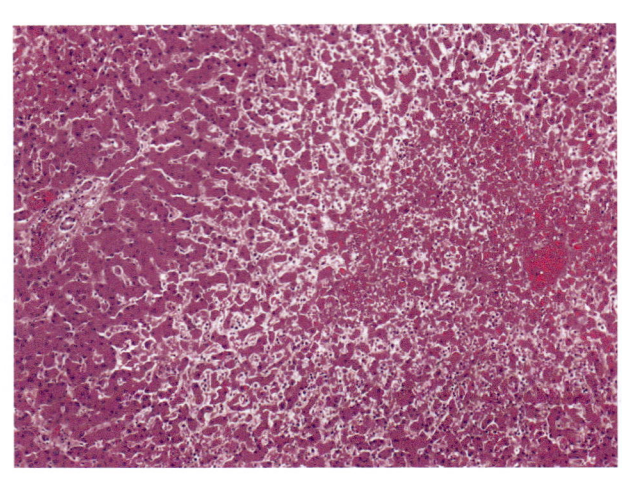

图1 肝细胞萎缩
Atrophy of liver
肝淤血,肝窦扩张,肝细胞受压迫体积变小

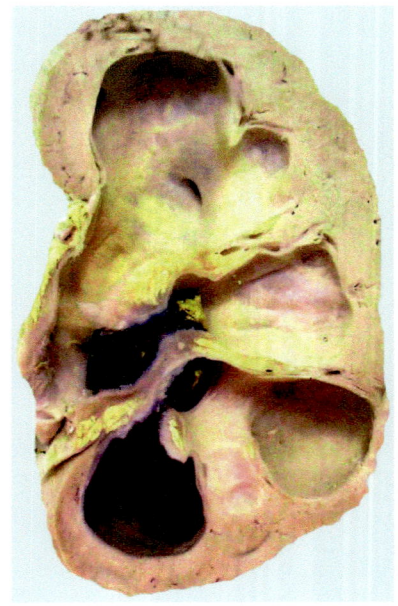

图2 肾压迫性萎缩
Pressure atrophy of kidney
肾盂输尿管移行处可见黑色结石,肾盂积水、扩张,肾实质受压变薄,皮、髓质分界不清

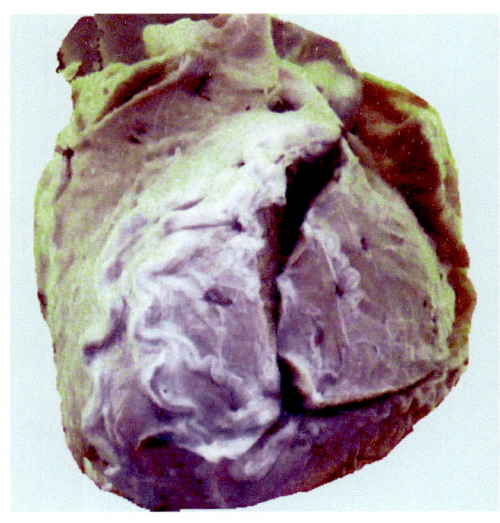

图3 心脏褐色萎缩
Brown atrophy of heart
心脏体积变小,重量减轻,色泽加深,冠状动脉分支因心脏变小而卷曲为蛇形弯曲

第1篇 病理学总论

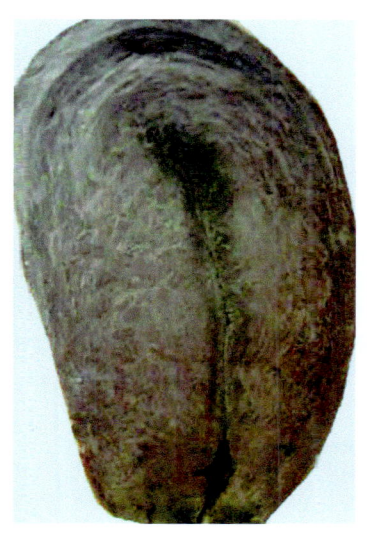

图4 子宫肥大
Hypertrophy of uterus
子宫体积增大，重量增加，肌壁增厚

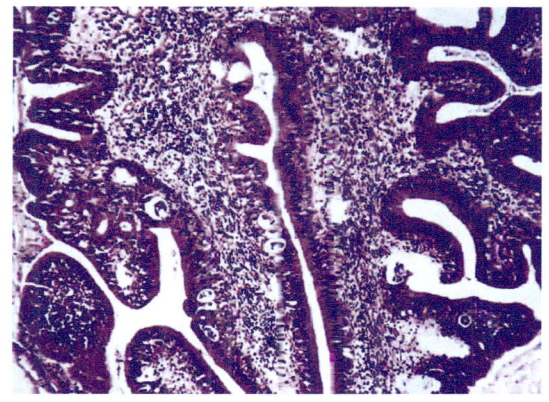

图5 鼻息肉腺体增生
Gland hyperplasia of polyp, nose

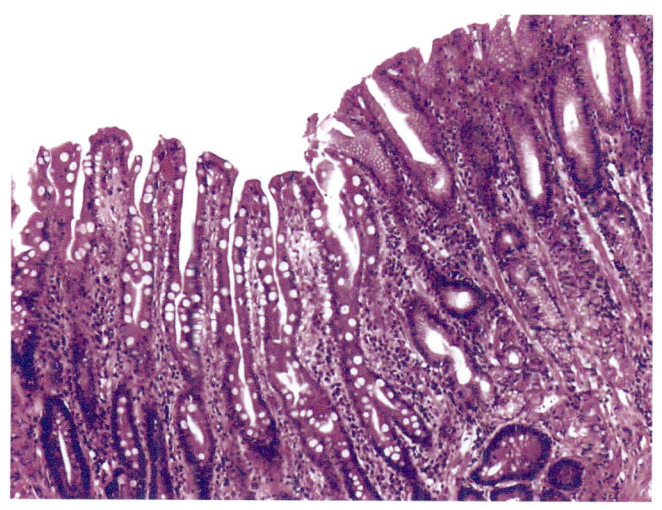

图6 胃黏膜肠上皮化生
Intestine metaplasia of stomach
胃黏膜腺体中出现大量肠黏膜中的杯状细胞，本例为慢性萎缩性胃炎

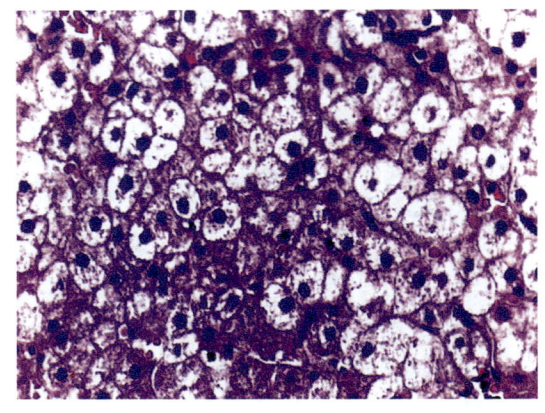

图7 肝细胞水肿
Cellular swelling of hepatocytes
肝细胞肿胀，胞浆空泡状、网状、疏松透亮，大者如气球状，为气球样变

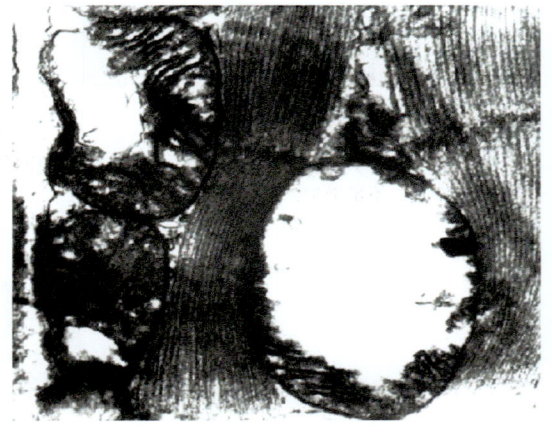

图8 心肌细胞水肿
Cellular swelling of myocytes
电镜下胞浆内线粒体肿胀，嵴变短、断裂

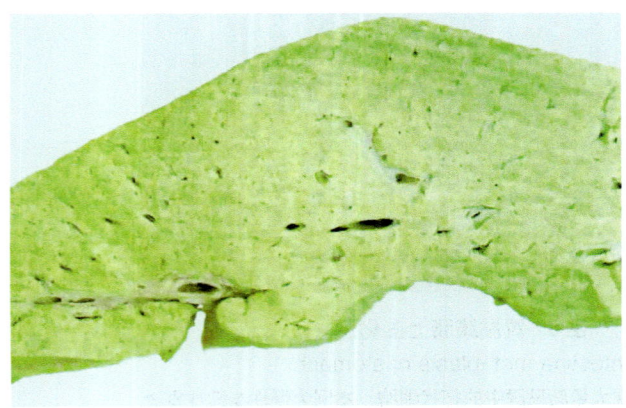

图9 肝脂肪变性
Fatty change of liver
肝额状断面，肝脏体积增大，呈弥漫性淡黄色，质软

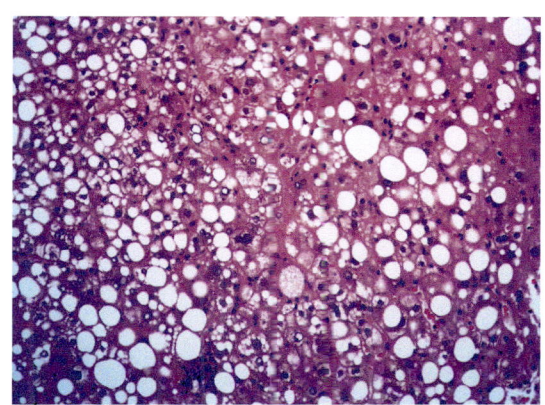

图 10　肝细胞脂肪变
Fatty change of liver
肝细胞胞质中见大小不等的圆形空泡（脂滴）

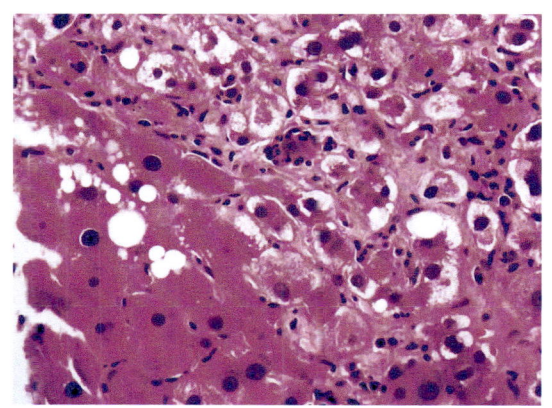

图 11　肝细胞玻璃样变
Hyaline degeneration of liver
左下方肝细胞胞质内呈均质红染状，为酒精性肝炎

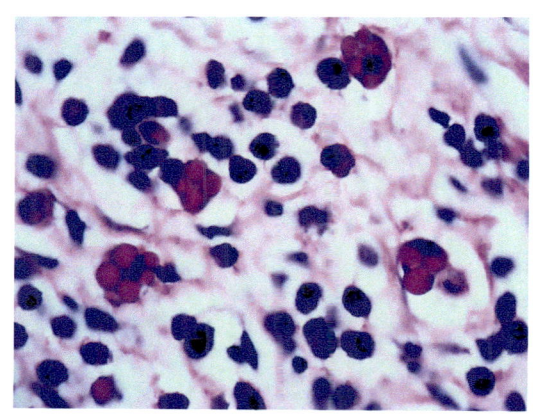

图 12　浆细胞 Rusell 小体
Rusell body of plasma cell
浆细胞内外见多个均质红染玻璃样小体

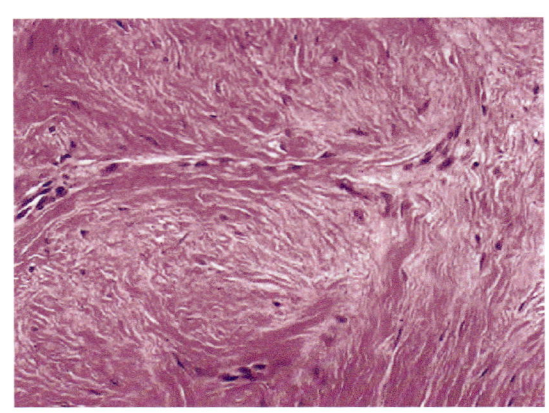

图13　纤维结缔组织玻璃样变
Hyaline degeneration of connective tissues
纤维细胞和血管大量减少，胶原增多，变粗，相互融合，呈红染均质状

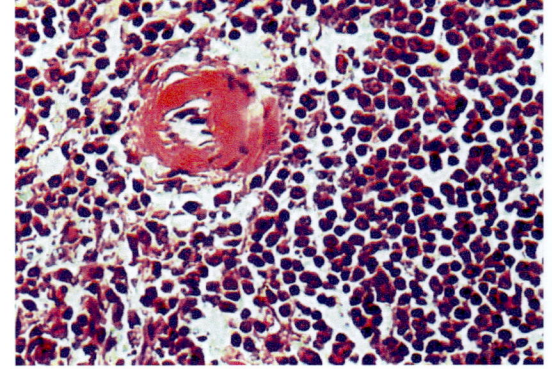

图14　脾中央动脉玻璃样变
Hyaline degeneration of spleen central arteriole
脾中央动脉壁厚，腔小，管壁呈红染、均质状

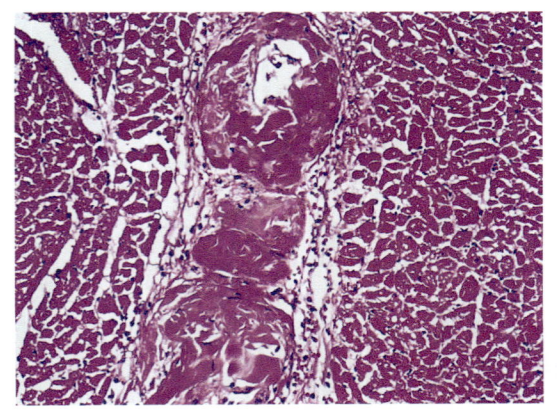

图15　心肌淀粉样变
Amyloidosis of heart
心肌间质小血管周围有淀粉样物质沉积，呈粉染团块状

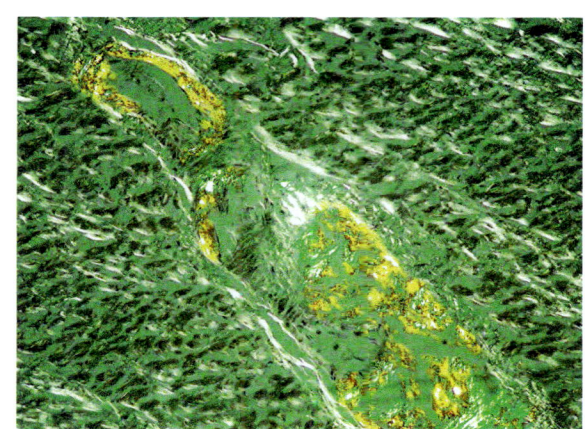

图16 心肌淀粉样变
Amyloidosis of heart
心肌间质小血管周围有淀粉样物质沉积，为刚果红染色，偏光显微镜观察

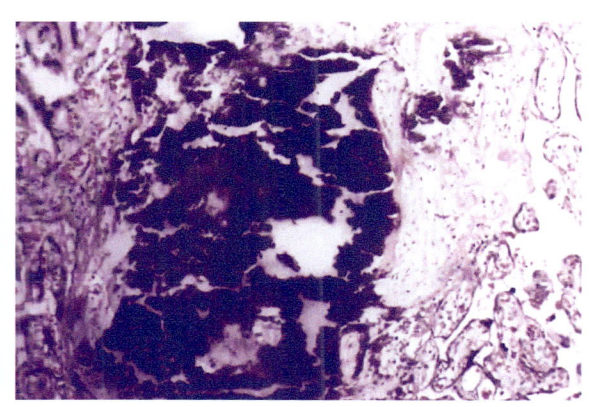

图17 胎盘钙化
Calcification of placenta
胎盘组织内呈蓝色的颗粒状钙盐沉积，为HE染色

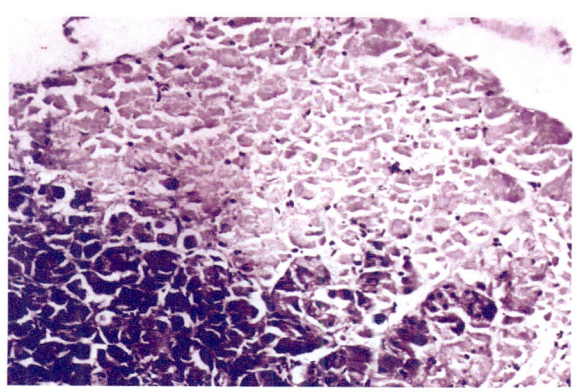

图18 胰腺凝固性坏死
Coagulative necrosis of pancreas
胰腺细胞坏死，核溶解消失，坏死组织粉染，胰腺组织结构轮廓存在

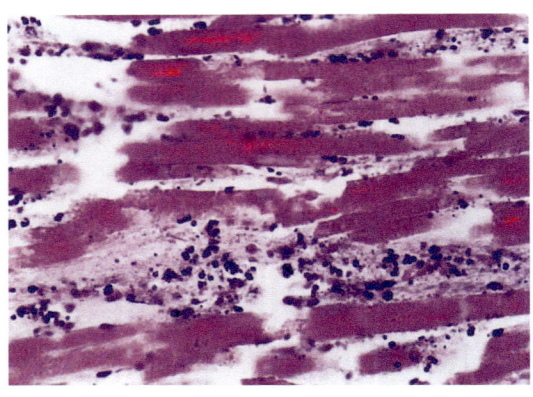

图19 心肌凝固性坏死
Coagulative necrosis of heart
心肌细胞核溶解消失，心肌纤维结构轮廓存在，心肌纤维间大量炎细胞浸润

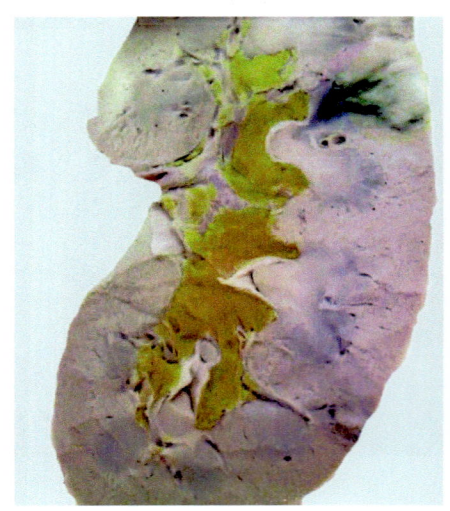

图20 肾凝固性坏死
Coagulative necrosis of kidney
肾冠状切面，梗死组织呈灰白色三角形，尖端指向肾门，底部向背膜，周围有充血出血带

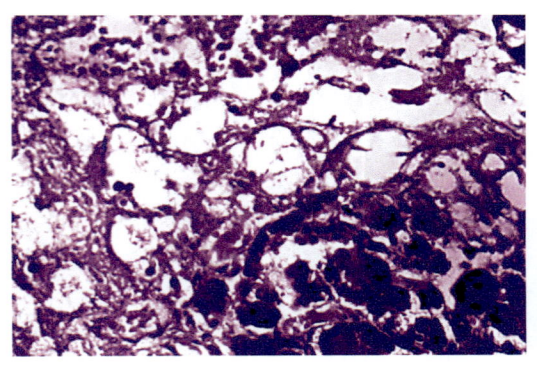

图21 胰腺液化性坏死
Liquefactive necrosis of pancreas
胰腺正常组织结构消失，细胞溶解液化

General Pathology 第1篇 病理学总论

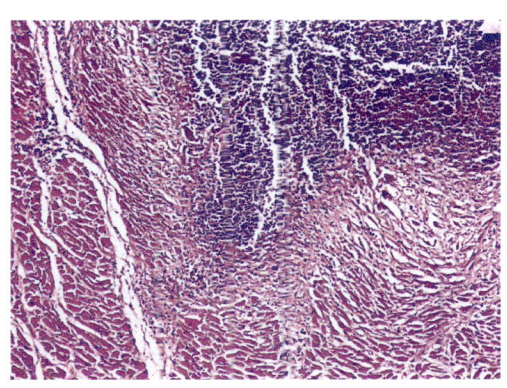

图22 心肌脓肿（液化性坏死）
Abscess of heart （liquefactive necrosis）
心肌局部组织坏死，大量中性粒细胞浸润形成脓液

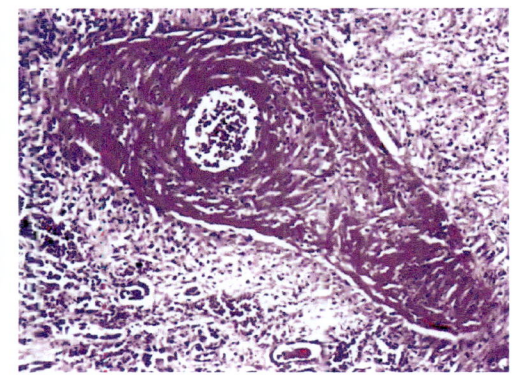

图23 动脉壁纤维素样坏死
Fibrinoid necrosis of artery
动脉壁正常组织结构消失，可见细丝状、颗粒状无结构红染物质

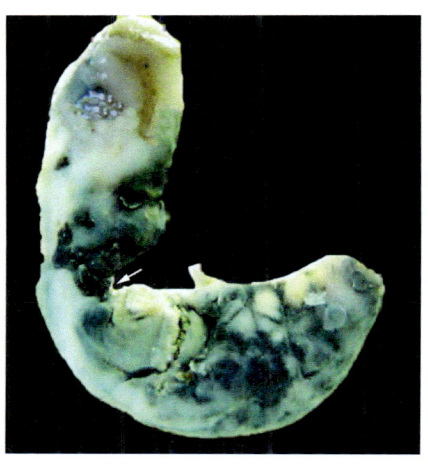

图24 阑尾湿性坏疽
Moist gangrene of appendix
阑尾肿胀坏死呈暗黑色，上部穿孔（图中白箭头示）

9

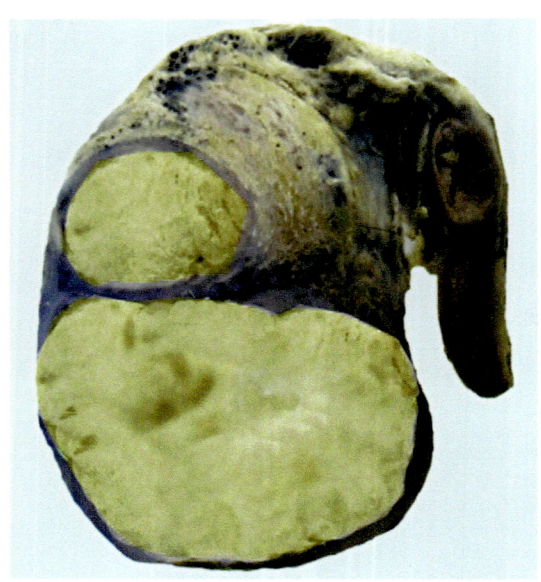

图25 淋巴结核干酪样坏死
Caseous necrosis of lymph node
淋巴结肿胀粘连成块，切面呈淡黄色，细腻，似奶酪样

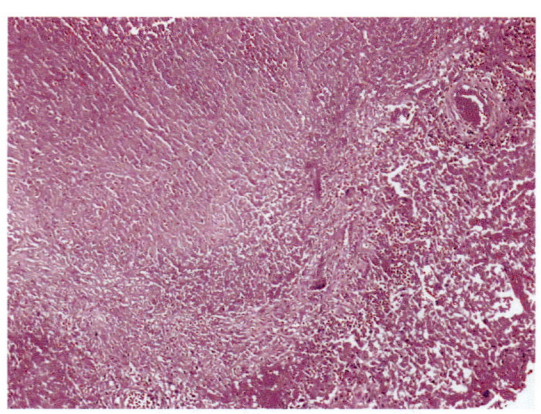

图26 淋巴结核干酪样坏死
Caseous necrosis of lymph node
淋巴结正常结构消失，可见红染、均质、无结构颗粒状物质

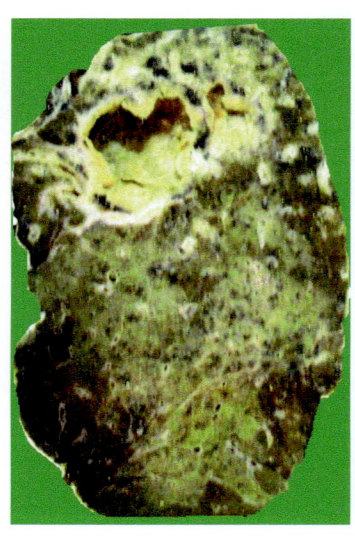

图27 肺结核空洞形成
Tubercular cavity of lung
肺结核干酪样坏死物分离排出，结核空洞形成

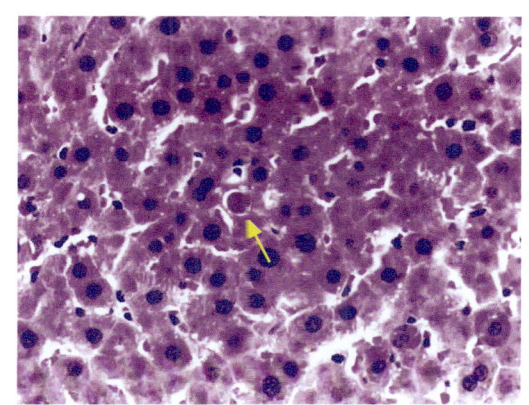

图 28 肝细胞凋亡
Apoptosis of liver
单个肝细胞凋亡（↑），与邻近细胞分离，形成球形嗜酸性小体

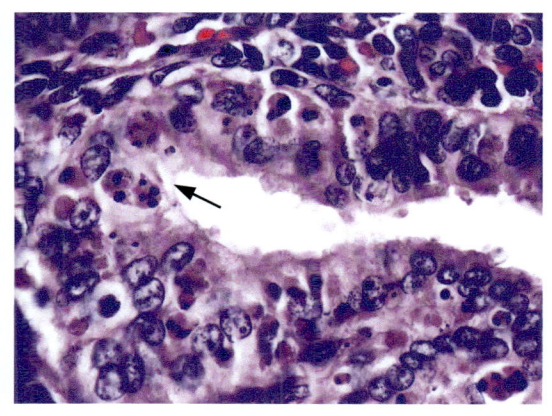

图 29 分泌期腺体的凋亡
Apoptosis of secretory gland
多个腺细胞凋亡（↑），与邻近细胞分离，胞质呈嗜酸性，核浓缩、碎裂

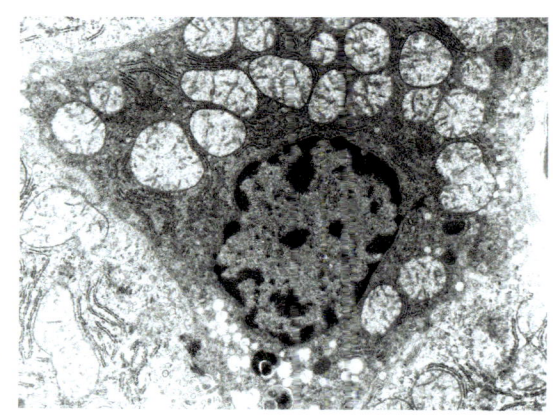

图 30 肝细胞凋亡
Apoptosis of hepatocytes
细胞皱缩，胞质致密，核染色质边集，膜结构完整

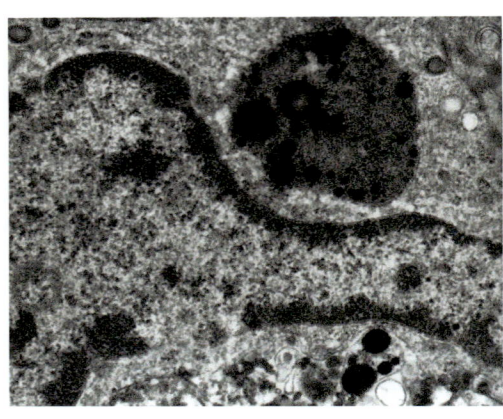

图31 巨噬细胞吞噬凋亡小体
Apoptosis body engulfed by macrophage
巨噬细胞包裹、吞噬凋亡小体

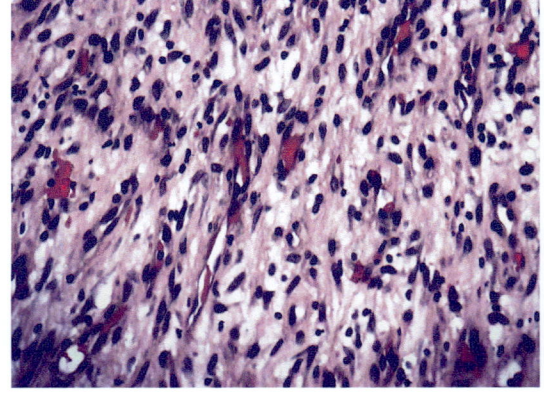

图32 肉芽组织
Granulation tissue
肉芽组织由新生毛细血管，增生的成纤维细胞和炎性细胞构成，毛细血管向伤口表面垂直生长

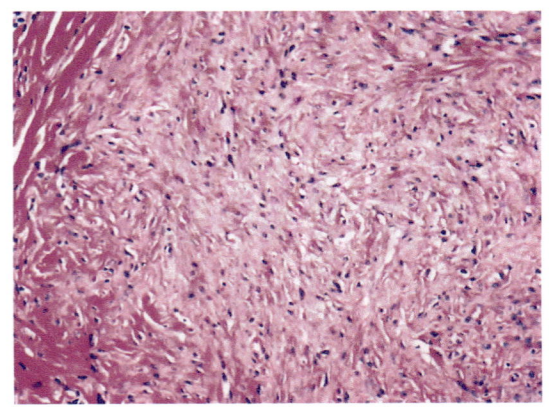

图33 瘢痕组织
Scar tissue
纤维细胞和血管减少，胶原增多，相互融合，呈均质红染状

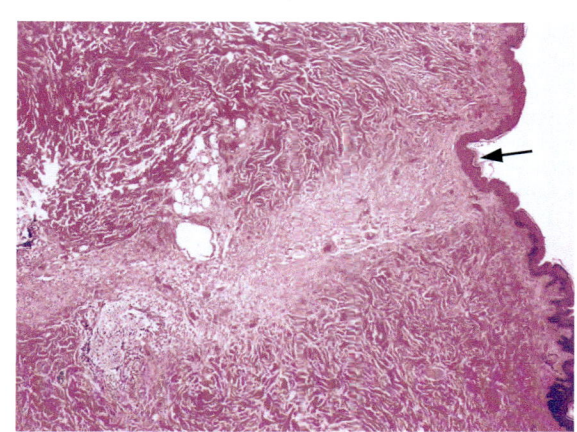

图34　Ⅰ期愈合
Healing by first intention
手术后Ⅰ期愈合伤口，皮肤刨缘
（↑）对合整齐，形成瘢痕小

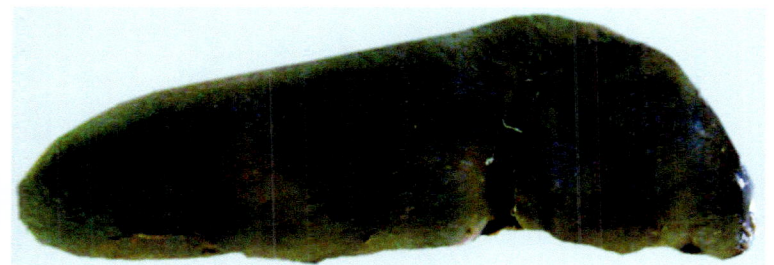

图35　脾淤血
Spleen congestion
脾脏体积增大，色暗红

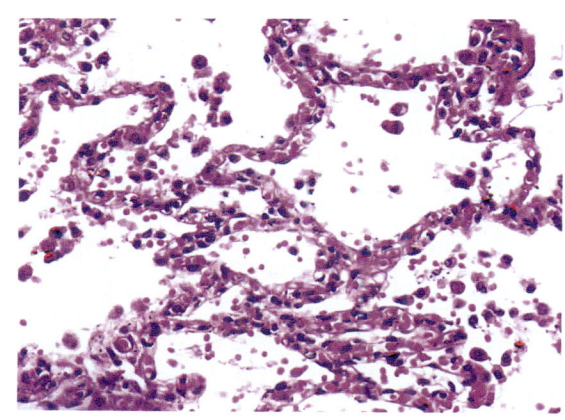

图36　肺淤血
Lung congestion
肺泡壁毛细血管扩张充盈，肺泡腔内
充满浅粉染水肿液

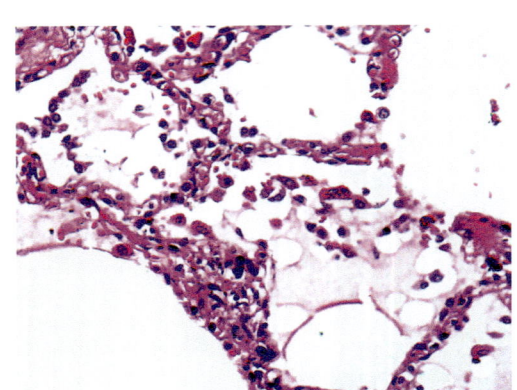

图37 肺淤血
Lung congestion
肺泡壁毛细血管扩张充盈，肺泡壁变厚，
肺泡腔内少量浅粉染水肿液及红细胞

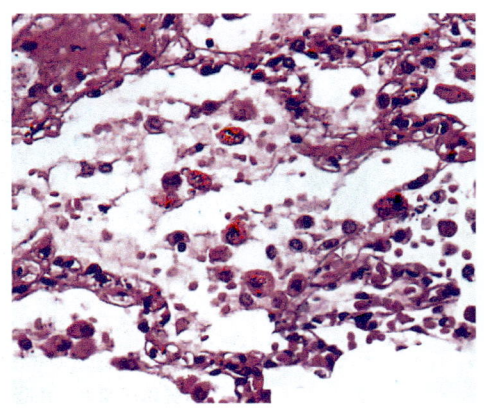

图38 慢性肺淤血（心衰细胞）
Chronic lung congestion（heart failure cells）
肺泡壁毛细血管扩张充盈，肺泡壁变厚，肺泡腔内有漏出红细胞，并可见含有含铁血黄素颗粒的巨噬细胞（心衰细胞）

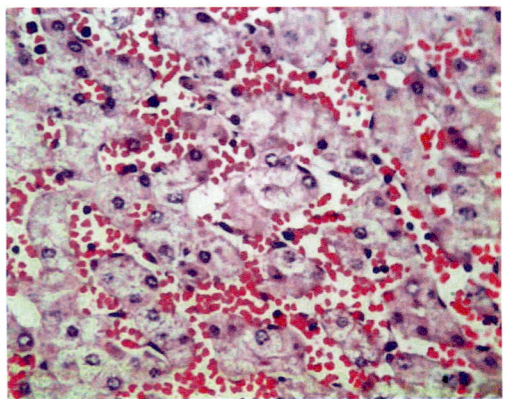

图39 急性肝淤血
Acute liver congestion
肝窦扩张，充满红细胞，肝细胞出现水样变性

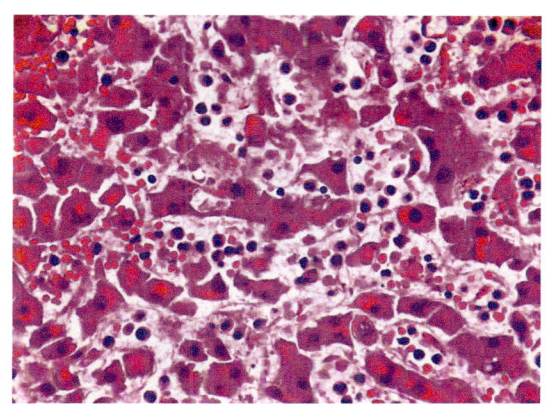

图40 慢性肝淤血
Chronic liver congestion
肝窦高度扩张淤血出血，肝细胞萎缩，甚至坏死消失

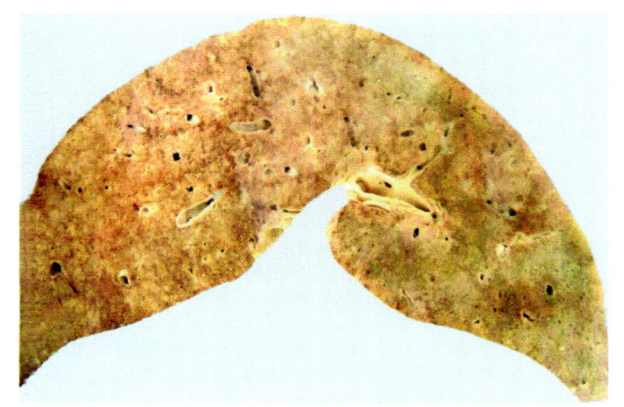

图41 槟榔肝
Nutmeg liver
慢性肝淤血，肝切面可见红（淤血）黄（脂肪变）相间的条纹，形似槟榔切面

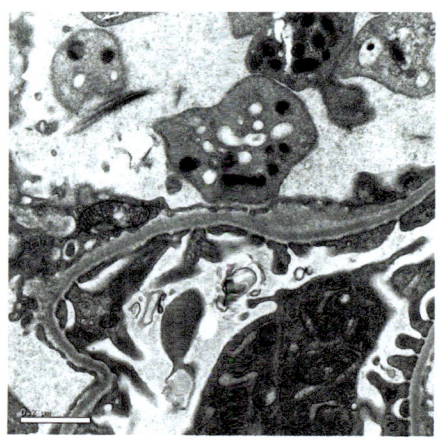

图42 血栓形成－血小板黏附
Thrombosis-platelets adhesion
电镜下观察在血栓形成初期，血小板黏附于血管内皮细胞表面

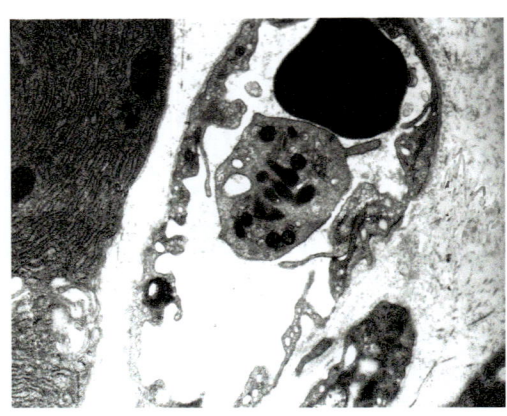

图43 血栓形成-血小板伪足
Thrombosis-pseudopod of platelet
血小板激活,可见伪足伸出

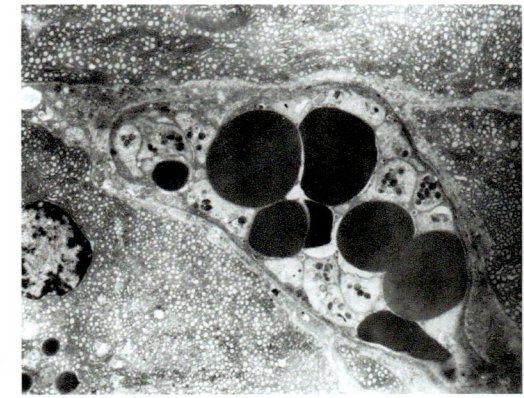

图44 血小板性血栓
Platelet thrombus
血小板不断黏集形成血小板性血栓

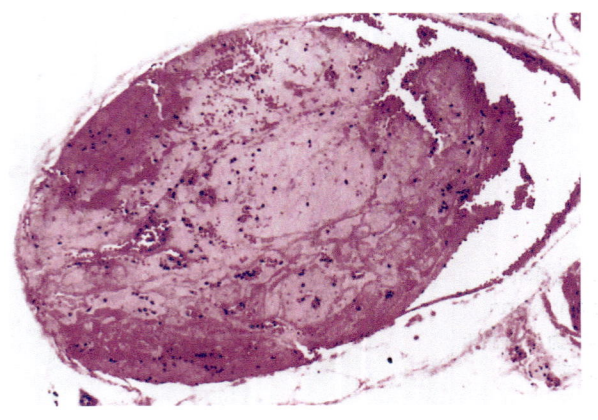

图45 白色血栓
Pale thrombus
镜下见白色血栓主要由粉染均质
的血小板和少量纤维蛋白构成

第1篇 病理学总论

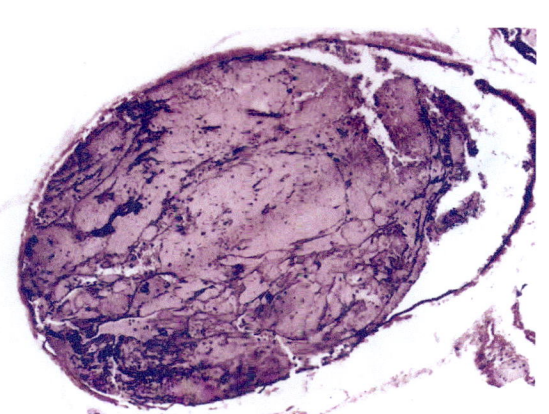

图46 白色血栓（PTAH 染色，同图 45）
Pale thrombus (PTAH staining, same as figure 45)
白色血栓中的纤维蛋白被染成蓝色丝状

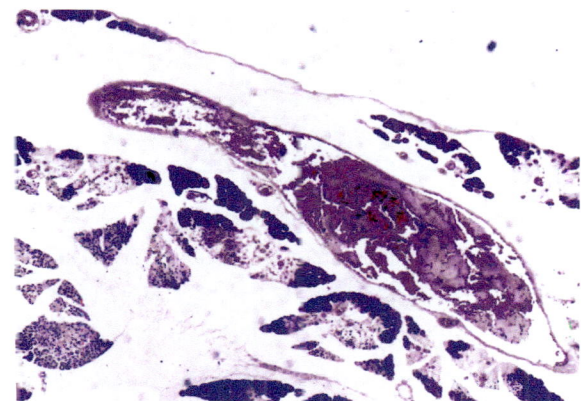

图47 胰腺小叶间动脉混合血栓
Mixed thrombus of artery in pancreas
血小板小梁之间可见血液凝固，充满大量红细胞和纤维蛋白

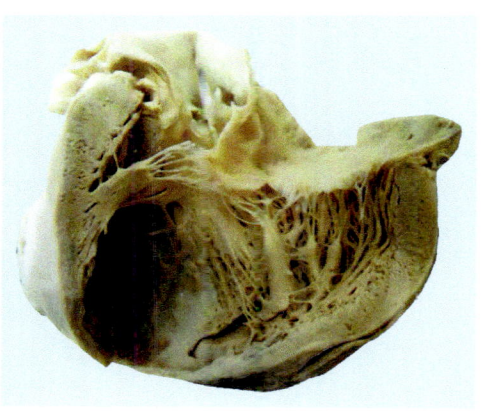

图48 心脏室壁瘤伴附壁血栓形成
Ventricular aneurysm with mural thrombosis
室壁瘤内侧可见灰褐色层状血栓黏附

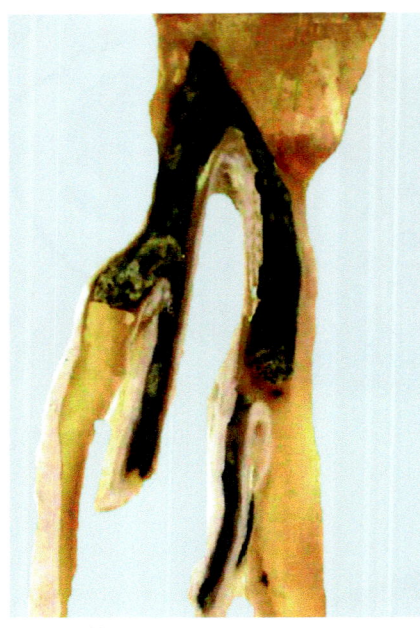

图 49　动脉内混合血栓
Mixed thrombus of artery
动脉壁可见动脉粥样硬化斑块，腔内可见灰白色和红褐色层状交替结构的血栓，呈粗糙干燥圆柱状

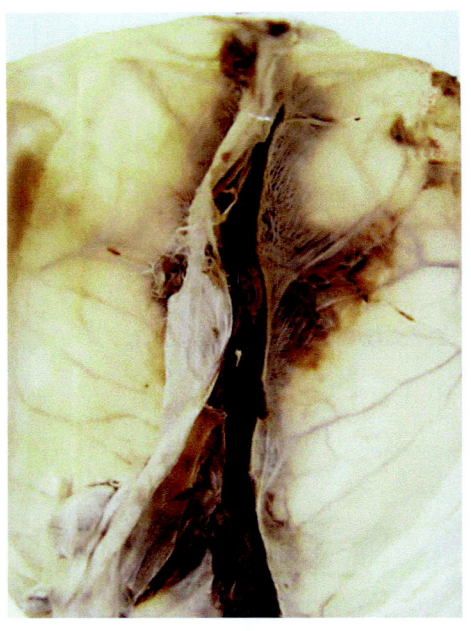

图 50　脑膜血管内血栓
Thrombus of meningeal blood vessel
脑膜血管内见一固体质块，灰褐相间，与血管壁粘连

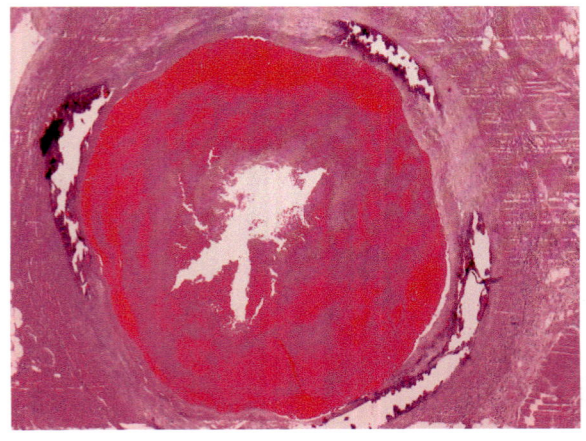

图 51　动脉内混合血栓
Mixed thrombus of artery
镜下见动脉管腔内血小板成梁状结构，血小板小梁之间是凝固的血液

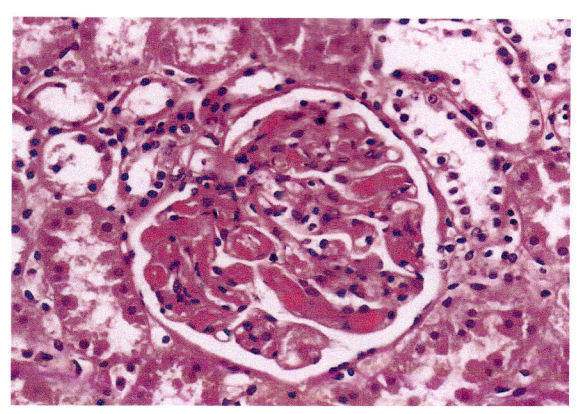

图52 DIC 肾小球毛细血管内微血栓形成
Microthrombosis of glomerulus during DIC
HE 染色见肾小球毛细血管内出现嗜酸性同质性物质

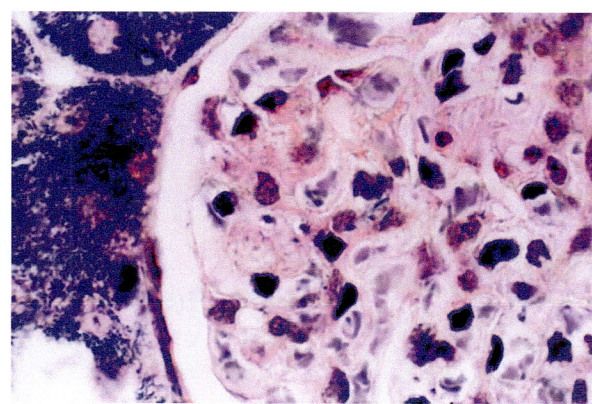

图53 肾小球内微血栓形成（PTAH 染色）
Microthrombosis of glomerulus (PTAH staining)
肾小球毛细血管腔内出现丝状或团块状蓝染物

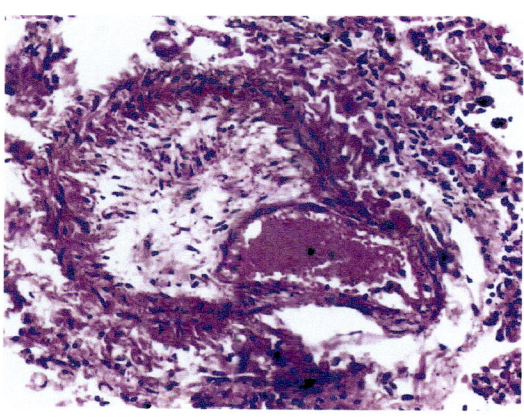

图54 血栓机化再通
Thrombus organization and recanalization
血栓左侧与血管壁连接紧密，并可见肉芽组织长入血栓内部，有新生血管形成

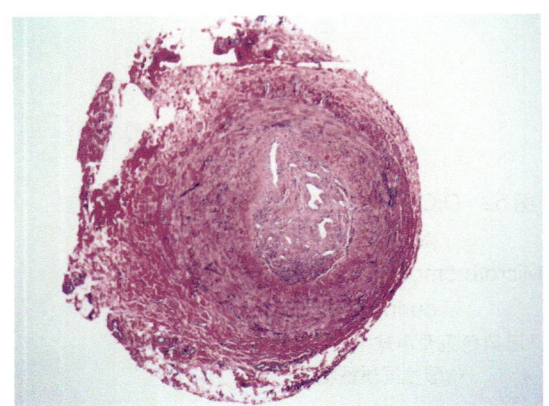

图55　血栓再通
Thrombus recanalization
血栓已发生机化，内部可见新生血管形成，使血流部分恢复

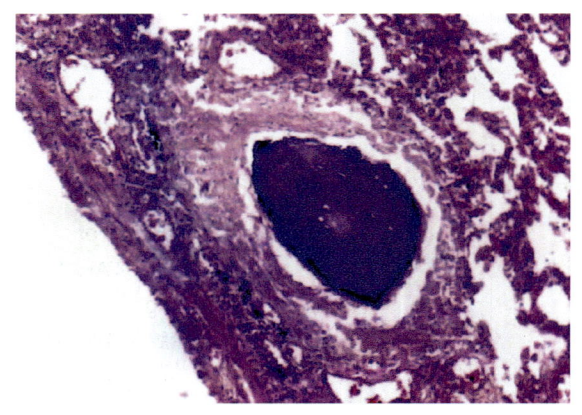

图56　血栓钙化
Thrombus calcification
血栓内可见蓝色团块状钙盐沉积

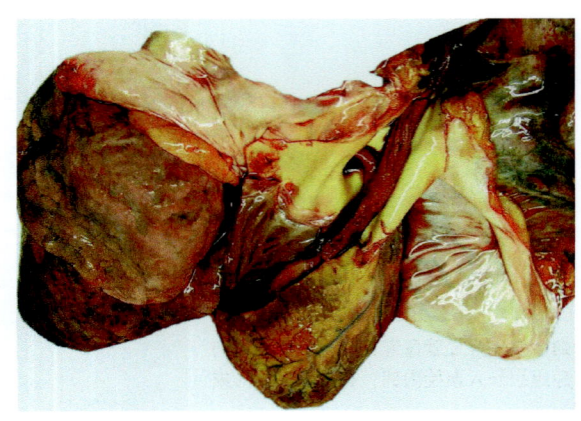

图57　肺动脉血栓栓塞
Pulmonary thromboembolism
肺动脉内可见一骑跨性血栓，从右心室一直延续到左右肺动脉主干，呈灰白条纹状

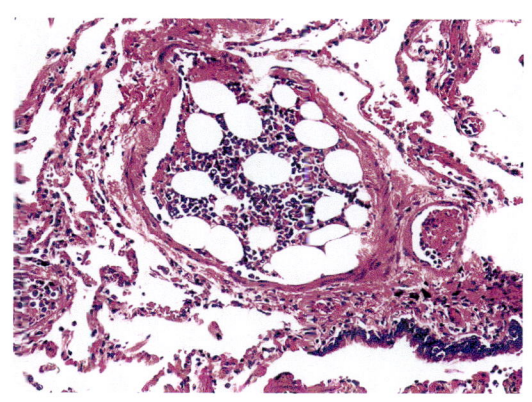

图 58　肺血管脂肪栓塞
Pulmonary fat embolism
肺血管管腔内可见骨髓细胞和脂肪滴

图 59　肾血管脂肪栓塞（胆固醇栓子）
Renal fat embolism (cholesterin embolus)
肾血管内可见呈针状裂隙的胆固醇结晶

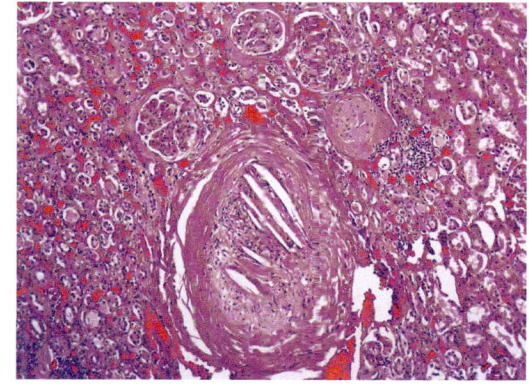

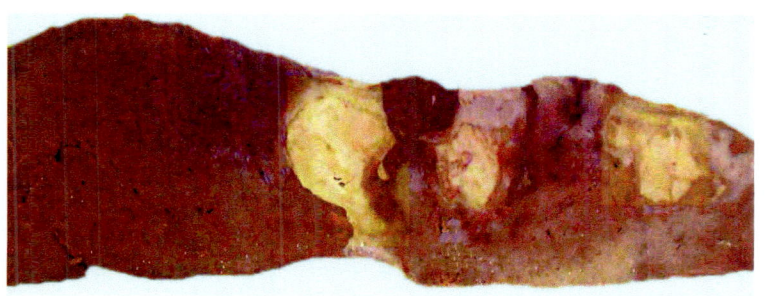

图 60　脾贫血性梗死
Anem c infarct of spleen
肉眼见脾梗死灶呈锥形，尖端指向脾门，底部靠近脾脏表面，梗死灶呈灰白色，周围有暗红色充血出血带

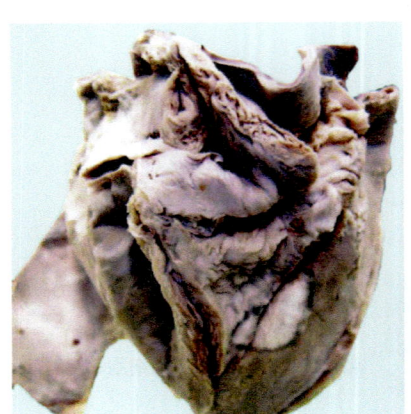

图 61 心肌梗死
Myocardial infarction
肉眼见心肌梗死灶呈不规则形,周围有暗红色充血出血带

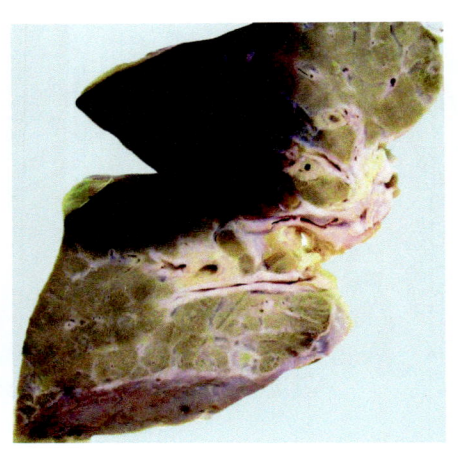

图 62 肺出血性梗死
Hemorrhagic infarct of lung
肉眼见肺梗死灶呈锥形,尖端指向肺门,底部靠近肺脏表面,梗死灶内大量出血,故呈暗红色

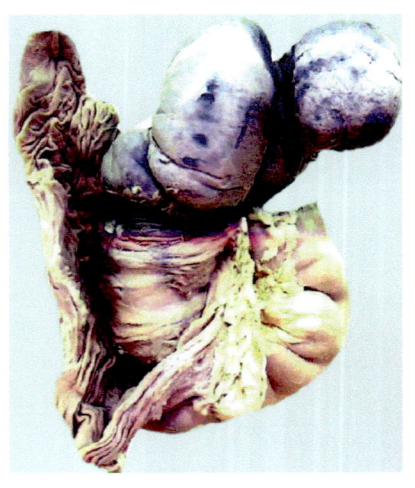

图 63 肠出血性梗死
Hemorrhagic infarct of intestine
肠套叠时,肠系膜的动静脉同时受压,造成肠壁的出血性梗死,梗死灶暗红色,呈节段性

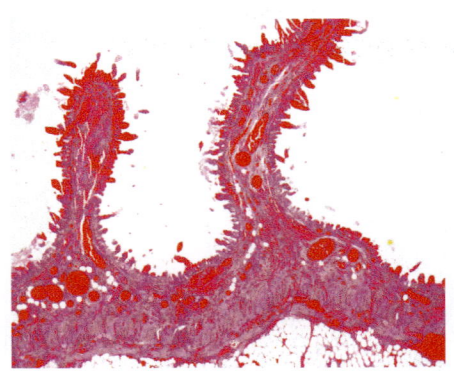

图 64 肠出血性梗死
Hemorrhagic infarct of intestine
镜下见肠壁坏死,坏死组织内大量出血,并见严重淤血

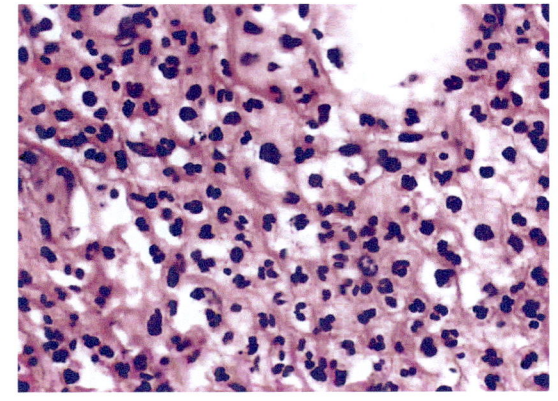

图 65　中性粒细胞
Neutrophil
细胞体积较小，胞浆淡粉染色，核呈分叶状

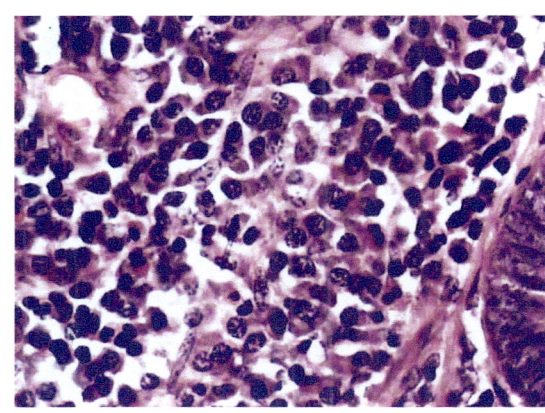

图 66　浆细胞
Plasma cell
细胞核圆形偏于胞体的一侧，染色质呈车轮状排列，胞质丰富略带嗜碱性，在核旁常形成空晕

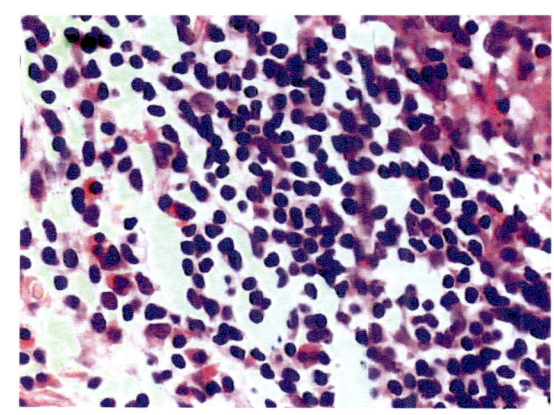

图 67　淋巴细胞
Lymphocyte
淋巴细胞体积较小，胞质极少，核圆形深染

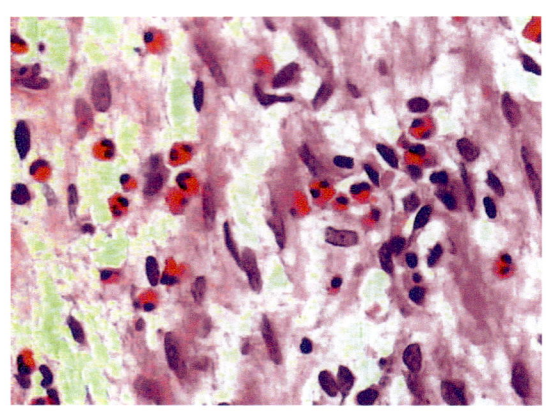

图 68 嗜酸粒细胞
Eosinophil
细胞核呈分叶状，胞质内含多量较大的嗜酸性颗粒

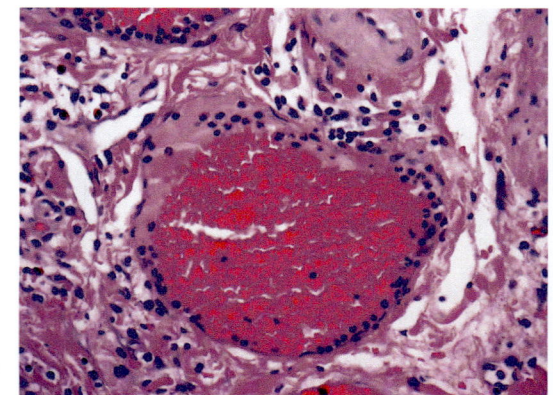

图 69 白细胞附壁
Leukocytic adhesion
白细胞黏附于血管的边缘部

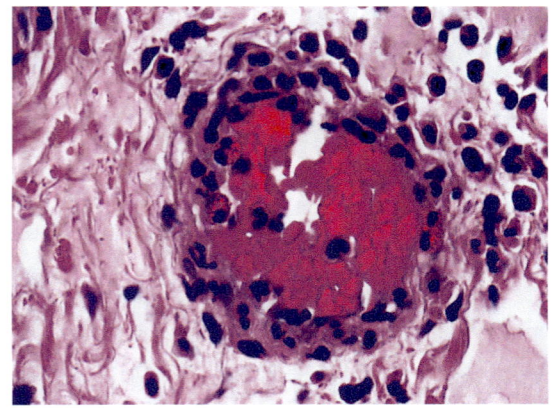

图 70 白细胞的游出
Leukocytic emigration
白细胞通过血管壁进入周围组织间隙

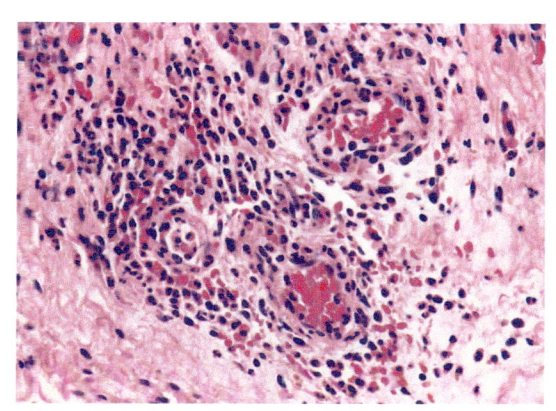

图71 红细胞的漏出
Red cells leak
白细胞的游出为主动过程;当血管壁严重损伤时有红细胞漏出,为被动过程

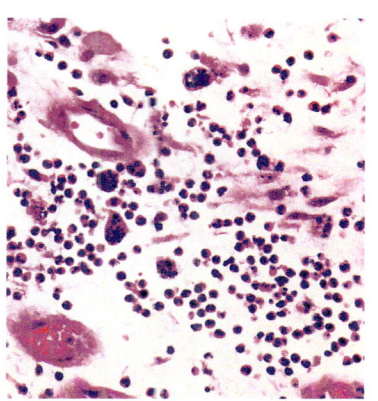

图72 白细胞的吞噬作用
Leukocytic phagocytosis
白细胞胞浆中可见吞噬的异物

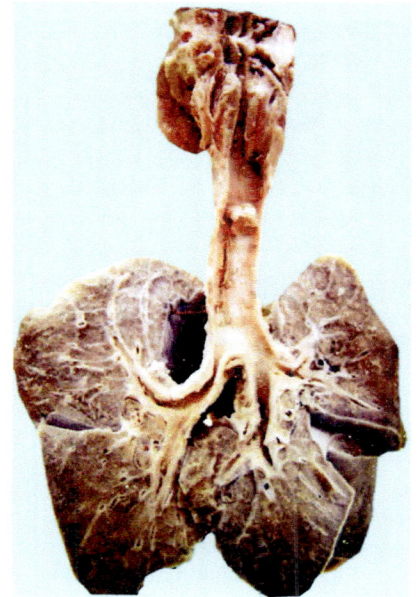

图73 气管纤维素性炎
Fibrinous inflammation of trachea
气管黏膜表面可见灰白色膜样结构

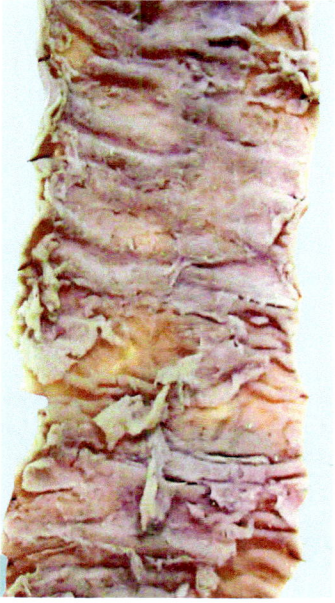

图74 肠纤维素性炎
Fibrinous inflammation of intestine
肠黏膜表面可见灰白色膜样结构

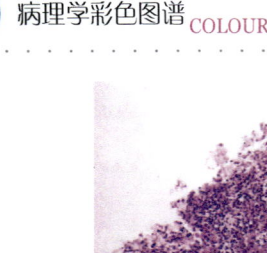

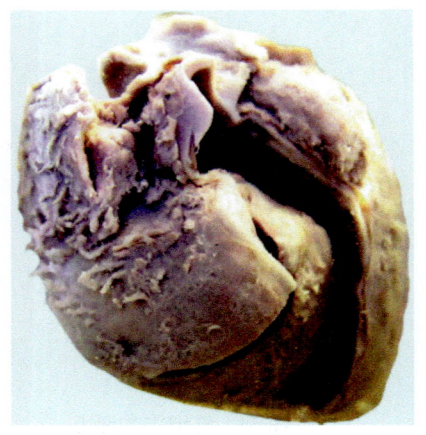

图 75　肠纤维素性炎
Fibrinous inflammation of intestine
肠黏膜表面可见渗出的大量纤维素，及坏死组织、炎细胞和红细胞

图 76　纤维素性心外膜炎
Fibrinous pericarditis
心包脏层可见灰白色绒毛样物质

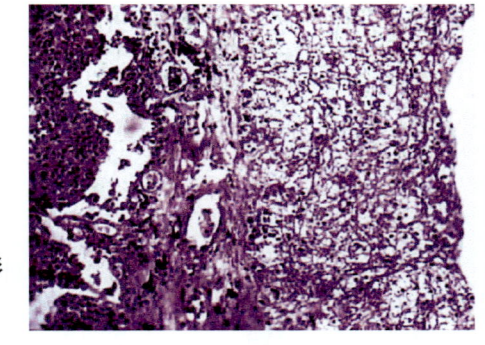

图 77　胸膜纤维素性炎
Fibrinous inflammation of pleura
胸膜表面大量的纤维素性渗出物，在纤维素形成的网眼中还可见渗出的炎细胞

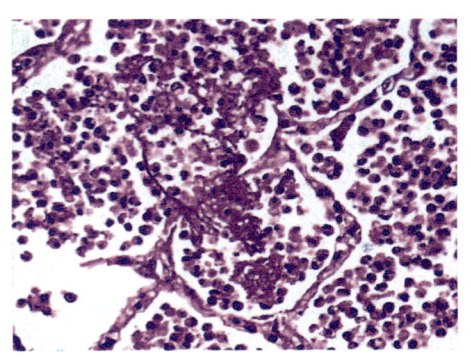

图 78　肺纤维素性炎
Fibrinous inflammation of lung
肺泡腔内可见大量渗出的纤维蛋白及中性粒细胞。相邻肺泡腔内纤维蛋白通过肺泡间孔彼此相连

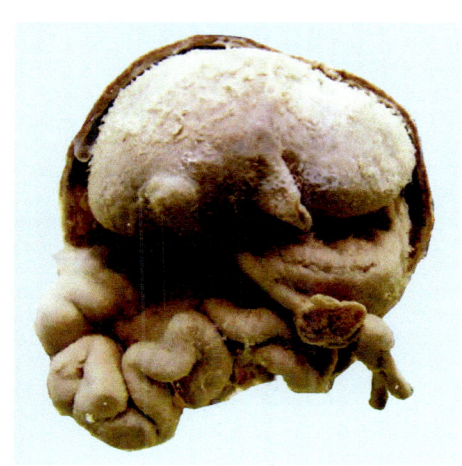

图 79 化脓性腹膜炎
Suppurative peritonitis
腹膜表面可见一层灰白色的脓膜

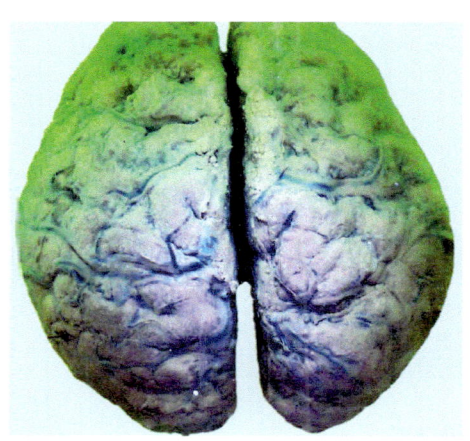

图 80 化脓性脑膜炎
Suppurative meningitis
脑膜表面覆盖了一层灰白色脓性渗出物
掩盖了脑表面的沟回

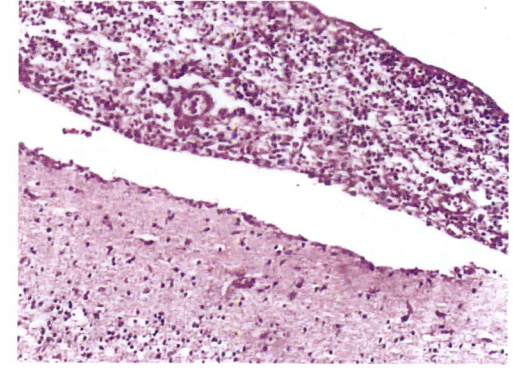

图 81 化脓性脑膜炎
Suppurative meningitis
大量的炎细胞渗出于蛛网膜下腔内，
脑实质未见明显病理学改变

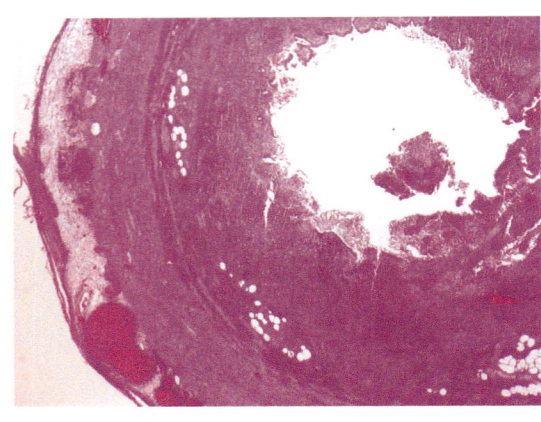

图82 急性蜂窝织炎性阑尾炎
Acute phlegmonous appendicitis
阑尾各层均见大量的炎细胞浸润

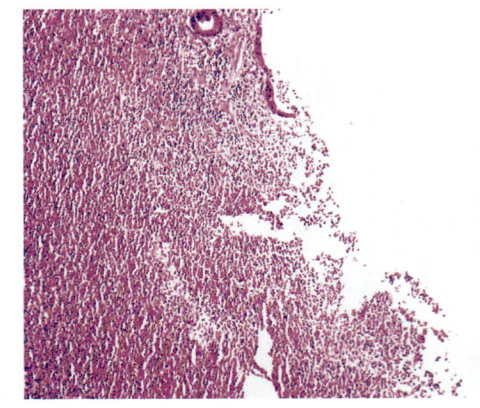

图83 急性蜂窝织炎性阑尾炎
Acute phlegmonous appendicitis
阑尾的黏膜层和黏膜下层大量炎细胞浸润，部分黏膜坏死脱落

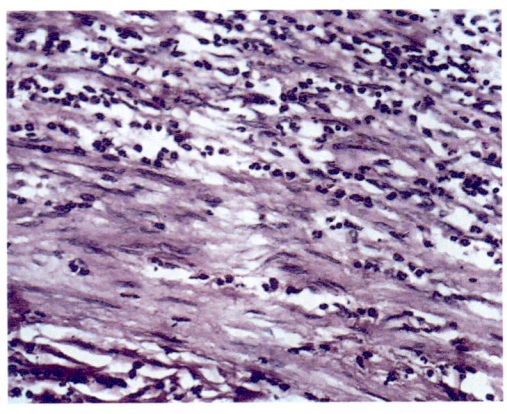

图84 急性蜂窝织炎性阑尾炎
Acute phlegmonous appendicitis
阑尾肌层疏松水肿，肌纤维间可见大量中性粒细胞弥漫浸润

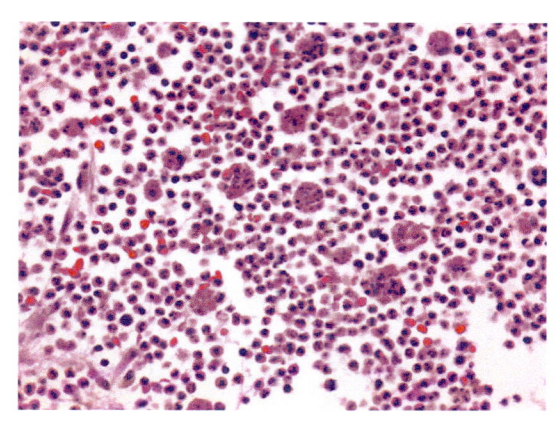

图 85 毛囊炎
Folliculitis
正常组织结构消失，大量中性粒细胞浸润，可见吞噬了坏死组织的巨噬细胞

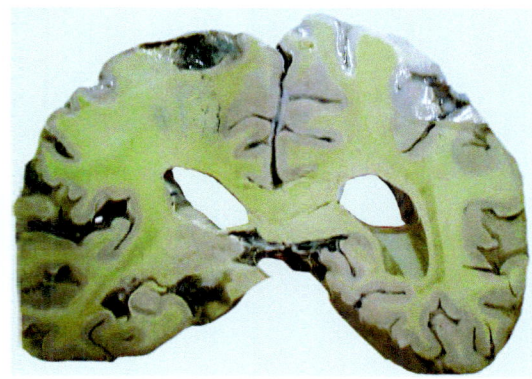

图 86 脑脓肿
Cerebral abscess
局部脑组织可见溶解坏死，形成充满脓液的腔

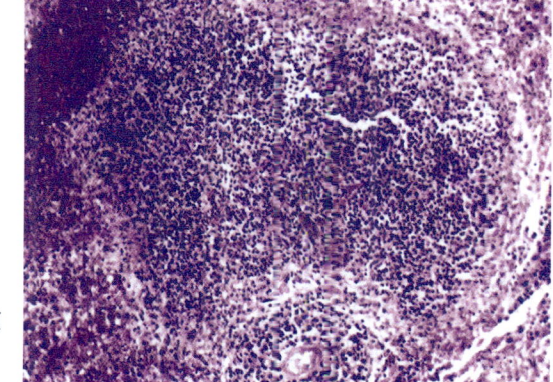

图 87 脓肿
Abscess
局部正常组织结构消失，可见红染颗粒状坏死组织和大量炎细胞浸润

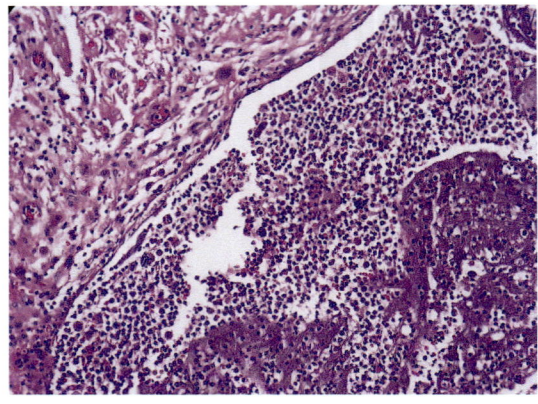

图 88 脓肿
Abscess
脓肿内组织完全坏死液化，可见脓肿腔内大量中性粒细胞浸润

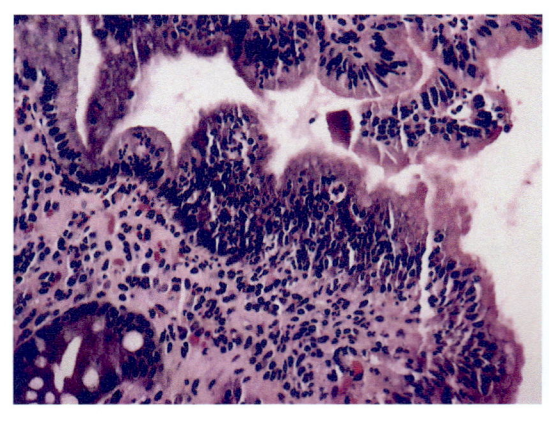

图 89 慢性胃炎
Chronic gastritis
胃黏膜及黏膜下层可见淋巴细胞、浆细胞及少量中性粒细胞的浸润。胃黏膜腺体可见肠上皮化生

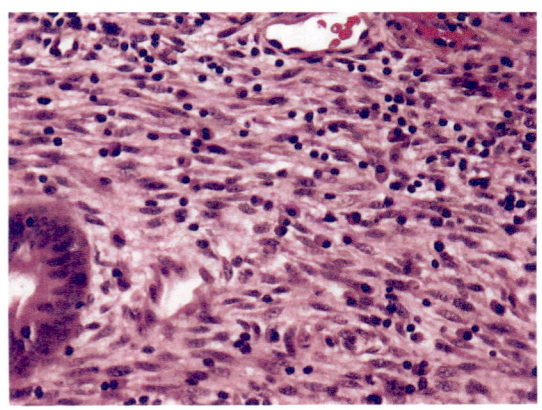

图 90 慢性子宫内膜炎
Chronic endometritis
子宫内膜可见浆细胞、淋巴细胞浸润

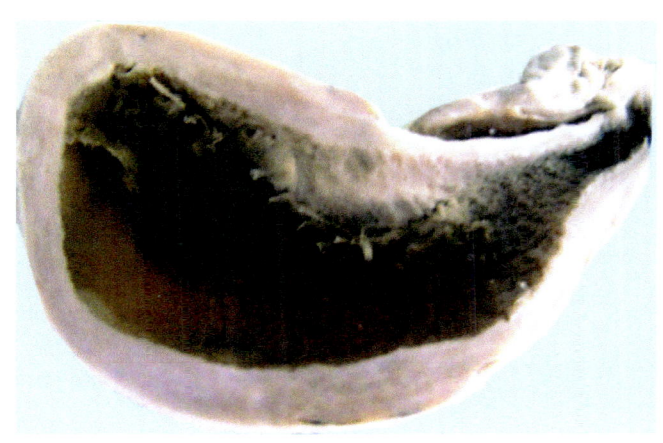

图 91　慢性胆囊炎
Chronic cholecystitis
胆囊壁增厚，灰白色，质地坚硬，黏膜萎缩，各层结构不清

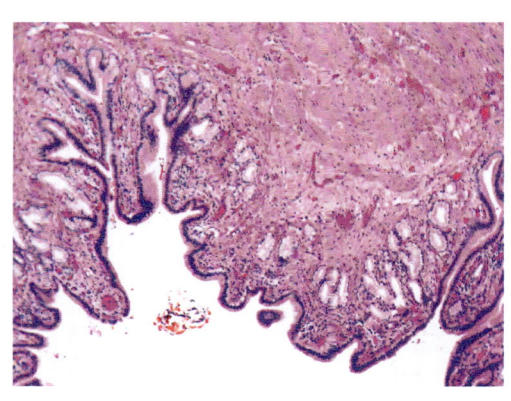

图 92　慢性胆囊炎
Chronic cholecystitis
胆囊黏膜发生萎缩，各层均有炎细胞浸润，
纤维化明显

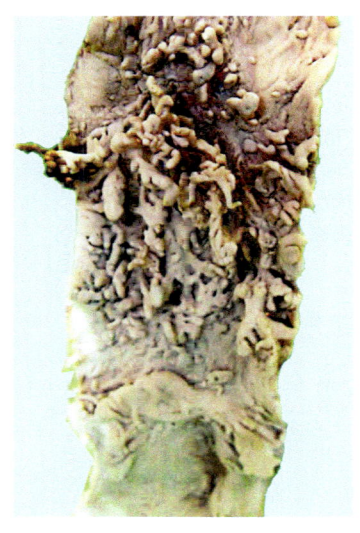

图 93　肠息肉
Polyp of intestine
肠黏膜面可见大小、形状不一的突起，互
相交织成珊瑚状，其基底与肠壁有蒂相连，
肠壁增厚，质地变硬

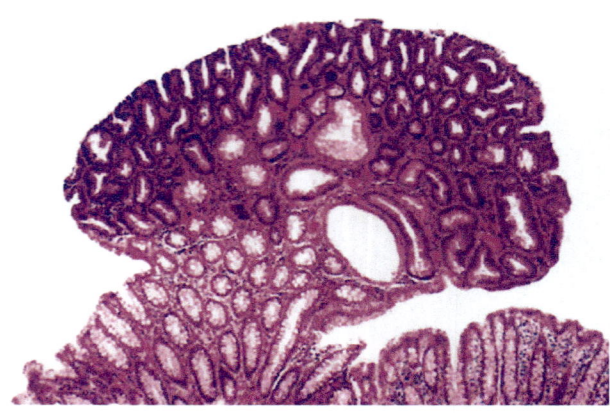

图94　肠息肉
Polyp of intestine
部分黏膜上皮、腺体及间质增生，间质内有大量炎细胞浸润

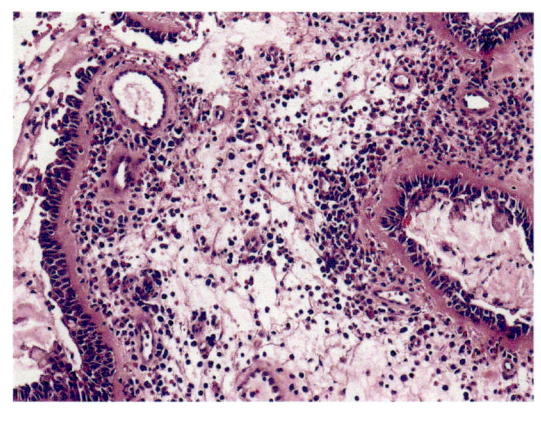

图95　鼻炎性息肉
Inflammatory polyp, nose
鼻黏膜上皮增生，鳞状上皮化生，黏膜下结缔组织增生，大量单核细胞、淋巴细胞、浆细胞、嗜酸粒细胞浸润

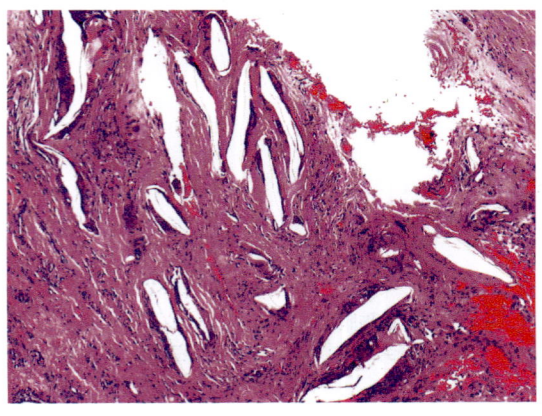

图96　异物肉芽肿
Foreign body granuloma
异物的长期刺激，形成慢性炎症。巨噬细胞增生，转变为上皮样细胞和多核巨细胞，围绕在异物周围

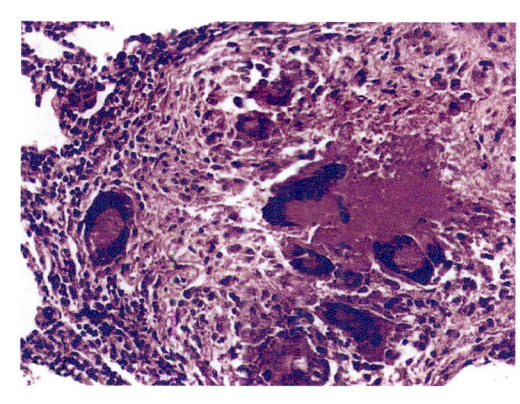

图 97　结核结节
Tubercle
结节中心为干酪样坏死，周围放射状排列上皮样细胞，并可见朗格汉斯巨细胞掺杂其中，再向外为大量淋巴细胞浸润，结核结节周围还可见纤维结缔组织包绕

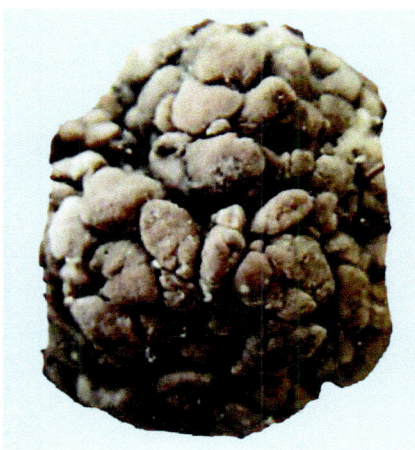

图 98　皮肤乳头状瘤
Papilloma of skin
肿瘤向表面呈外生性生长，形成许多指状、乳头状突起，呈菜花状或绒毛状外观，其根部狭窄成蒂与正常组织相连

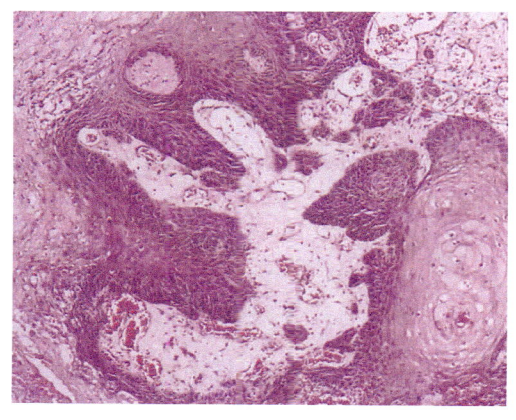

图 99　皮肤乳头状瘤
Papilloma of skin
肿瘤表面为增生的上皮，乳头轴心为较多血管的结缔组织间质（纤维脉管索）

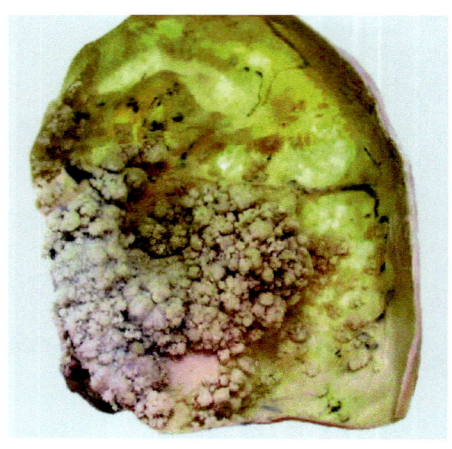

图100 卵巢浆液性囊腺瘤
Serous cystadenoma of ovary
输卵管下方附着一儿头大囊性肿物,表面光滑,灰白色,切面肿瘤呈单房性,囊内浆液已流出(为清亮透明的液体),囊壁不光滑,有乳头生长

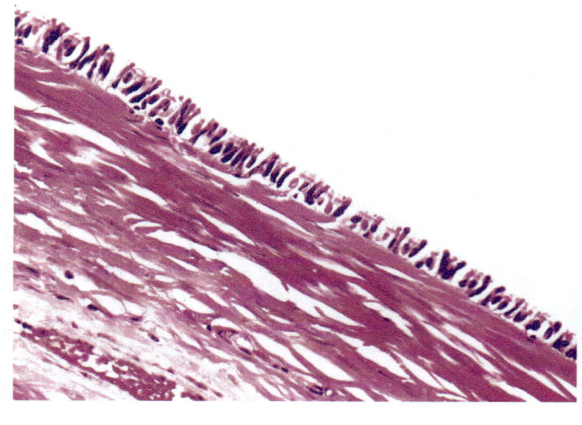

图101 卵巢浆液性囊腺瘤
Serous cystadenoma of ovary
囊腔被覆单层立方上皮,具有纤毛,与输卵管上皮相似

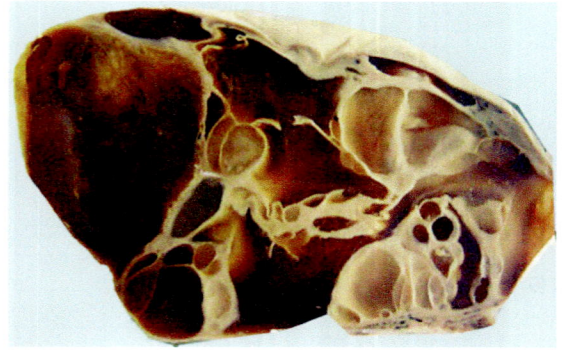

图102 卵巢黏液性囊腺瘤
Mucinous cystadenoma of ovary
儿头大小的囊性肿物,表面光滑,灰白色,切面肿瘤多房性,房壁薄如纸,灰白色,光滑湿润,囊腔内充以灰白色黏液

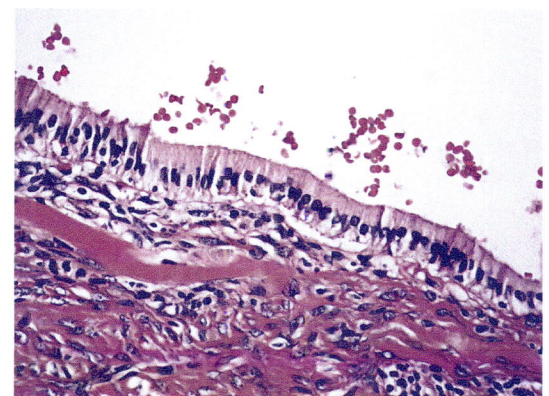

图 103 卵巢黏液性囊腺瘤
Mucinous cystadenoma of ovary
肿瘤囊腔被覆单层高柱状上皮,核位于基底部,核上方充满黏液

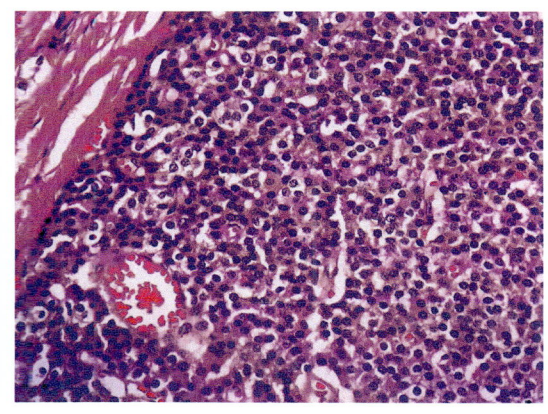

图 104 甲状旁腺腺瘤
Parathyroid adenoma
肿瘤边界清楚,细胞丰富,排列成实体片状。由主细胞、透明细胞和嗜酸性细胞混合而成

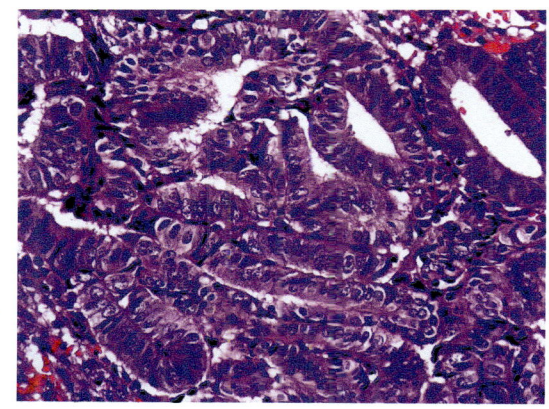

图 105 子宫内膜非典型性增生
Endometrial atypical hyperplasia
子宫内膜腺体明显增生,排列拥挤,上皮细胞呈轻至中度异型

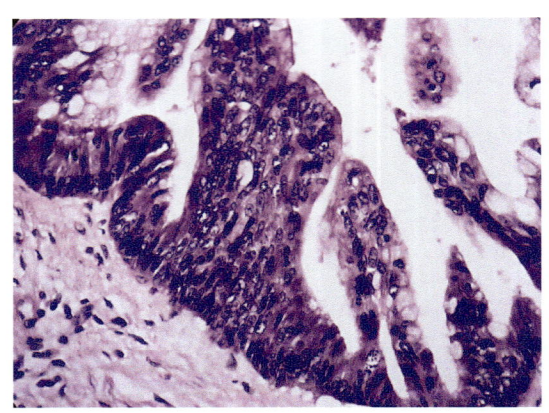

图 106　胰腺原位癌
Carcinoma in situ of pancreas
癌细胞累及上皮全层，尚未突破基底膜

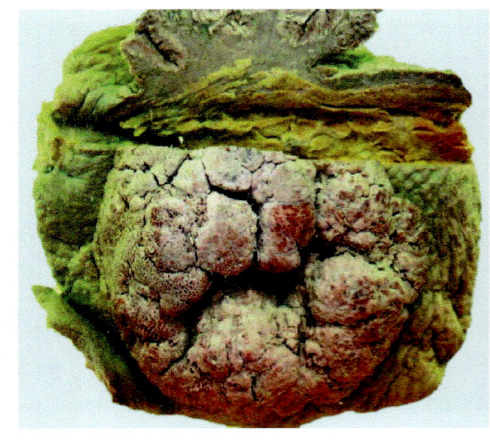

图 107　皮肤鳞癌
Squamous carcinoma of skin
皮肤表面有灰白色肿物，"火山口"状溃疡，肿瘤无包膜，表面干燥，较硬，灰白色。切面呈树根状浸润生长

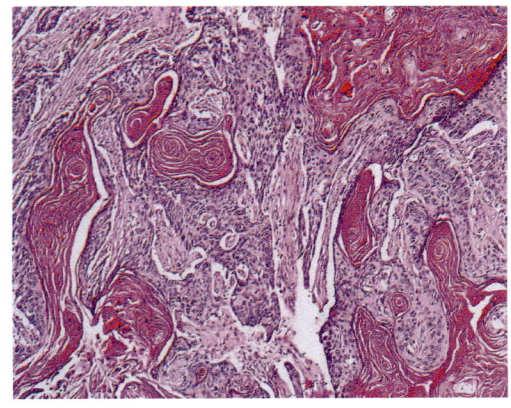

图 108　高分化鳞癌
Well differentiated squamous carcinoma
癌细胞形成不规则或条索状癌巢，分化较好，癌巢中央可出现层状的角化物，称为角化珠或癌珠

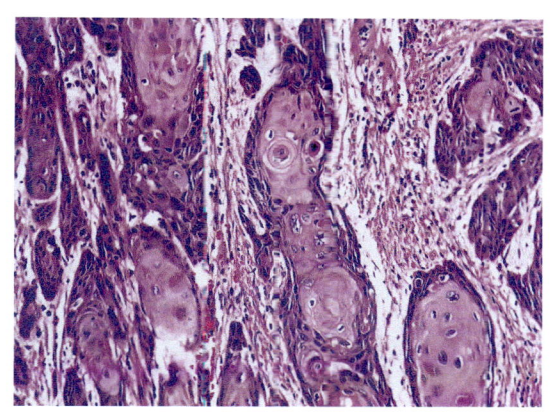

图109 直肠肛门鳞癌
Squamous carcinoma of rectum
镜下可见增生的上皮突破基底膜向深层浸润，形成条索状癌巢，癌巢中有相当于基底层的细胞，排列在癌巢的外层，其内为相当于细胞层的细胞

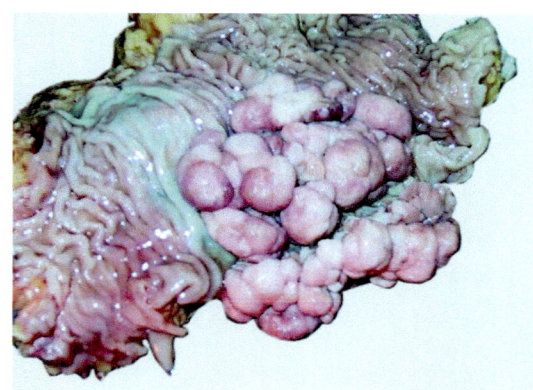

图110 结肠癌
Carcinoma of colon
已打开之结肠组织一段，肠腔内可见一约5cm×5cm大小肿块，向腔内突出，呈结节状生长，肿块呈灰粉色

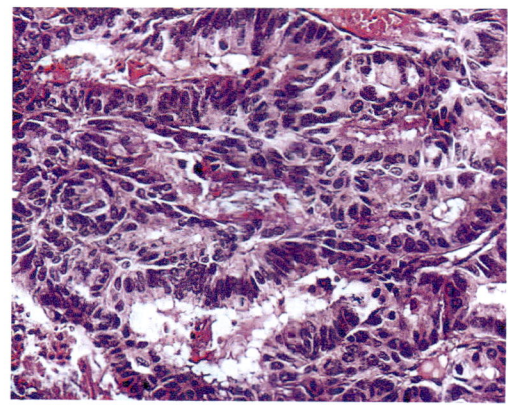

图111 结肠腺癌
Adenocarcinoma of colon
肿瘤组织排成不规则腺样结构，细胞层次增多，极向紊乱，可见"背靠背"和共壁现象，细胞异型性较明显

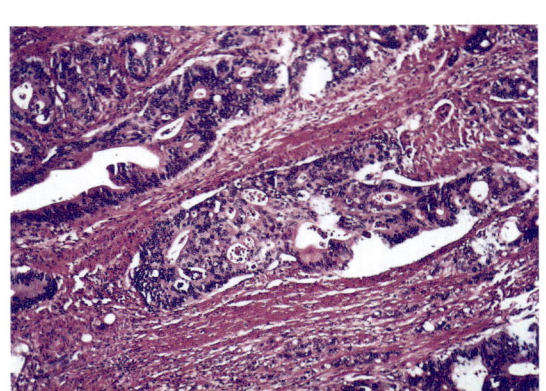

图 112 盲肠腺癌
Adenocarcinoma of cecum
肿瘤腺腔样结构高度不规则或缺如。腺腔有"背靠背"和共壁现象

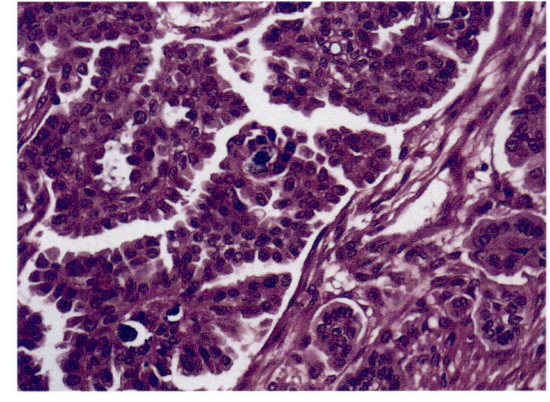

图 113 卵巢浆液性囊腺癌
Serous cystadenocarcinoma of ovary
肿瘤组织以乳头结构为主,乳头具有纤细的结缔组织轴心,肿瘤上皮呈立方形,可见砂粒体,少数区域呈腺样结构

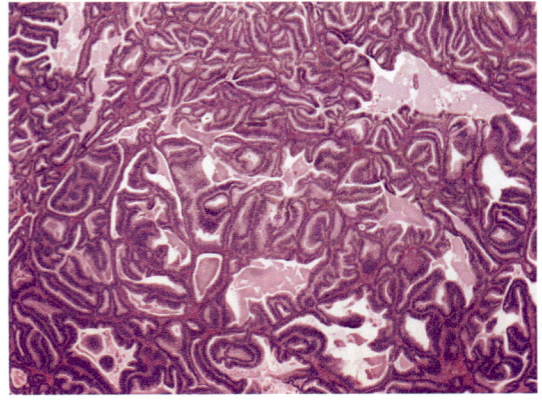

图 114 高分化子宫内膜样腺癌
Well differentiated endomertrioid adenocarcinoma
肿瘤由不规则的、复杂的管状腺体构成,腺体上皮细胞为立方型。管状腺体间由稀薄间质相互隔开,呈"背靠背"排列

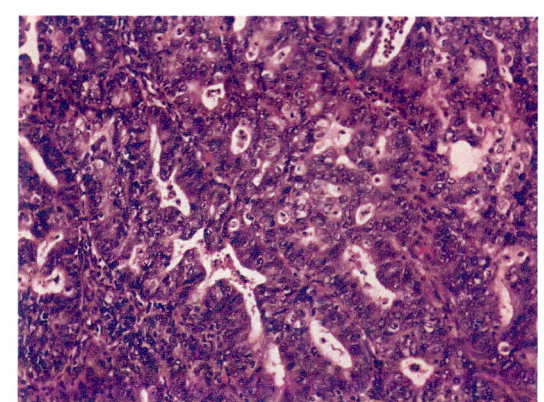

图 115 低分化子宫内膜样腺癌
Poorly differentiated endomertrioid adenocarcinoma
部分腺体实性结构，细胞的异型性显著

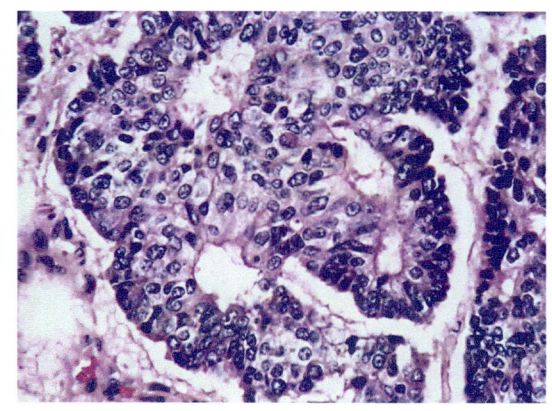

图 116 子宫内膜样腺癌
Endomertricid adenocarcinoma
增生的腺体排列紊乱，腺腔大小不一，形状不规则 并可见实性细胞团

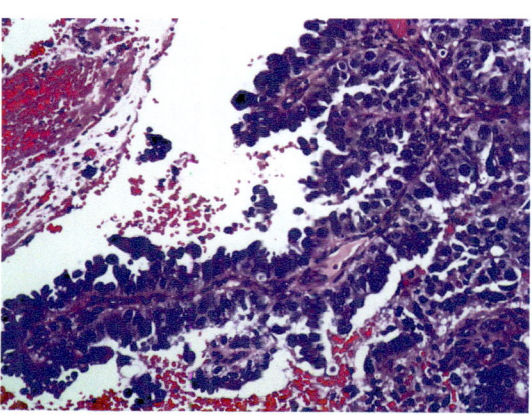

图 117 子宫内膜浆液性乳头状癌
Endomertrial serous papilary carcinoma
肿瘤组织以乳头结构为主，乳头具有纤细的结缔组织轴心。肿瘤细胞核大，异型性明显

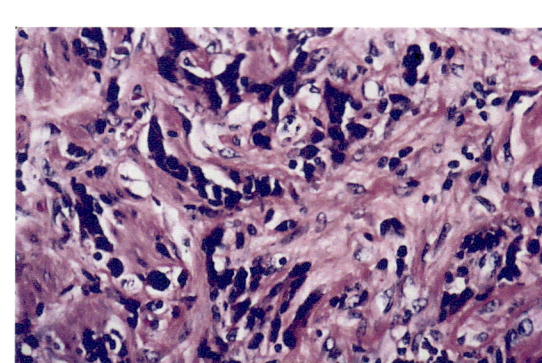

图 118　弥漫型胃腺癌
Diffuse adenocarcinoma of stomach
癌细胞呈索状或巢状排列，细胞体积小，异型性明显

图 119　胃印戒细胞癌
Signet-ring cell carcinoma of stomach
肿瘤细胞增生并弥漫浸润，瘤细胞分泌黏液于细胞内，使细胞核偏位呈印戒状

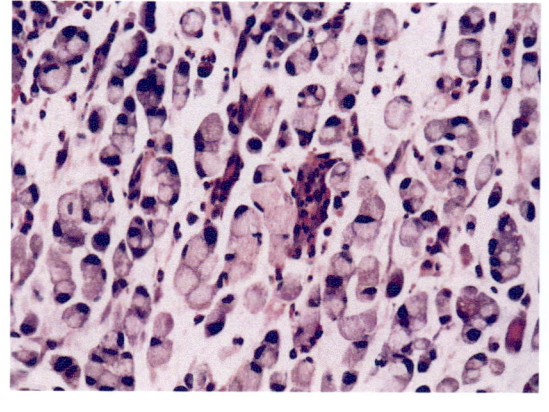

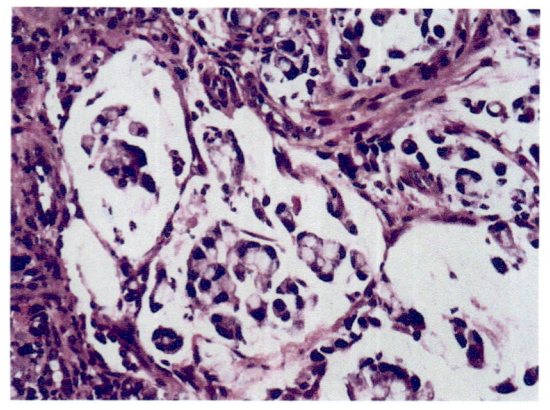

图 120　胃印戒细胞癌
Signet-ring cell carcinoma of stomach
肿瘤细胞增生并弥漫浸润，部分瘤细胞分泌黏液于细胞内，使细胞核偏位呈印戒状

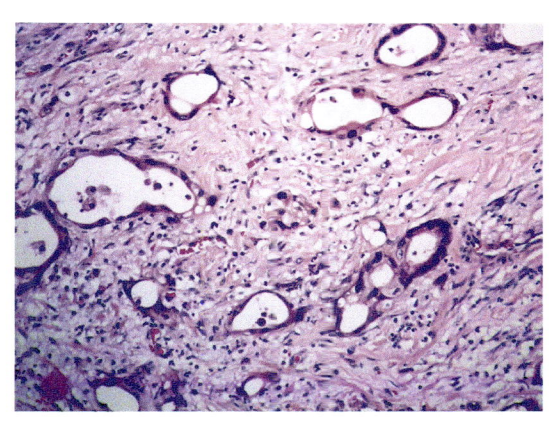

图 121 胰腺导管腺癌
Ductal Adenocarcinoma of pancreas
肿瘤细胞排列形成腺管样，腺腔不规则，其间有丰富的间质

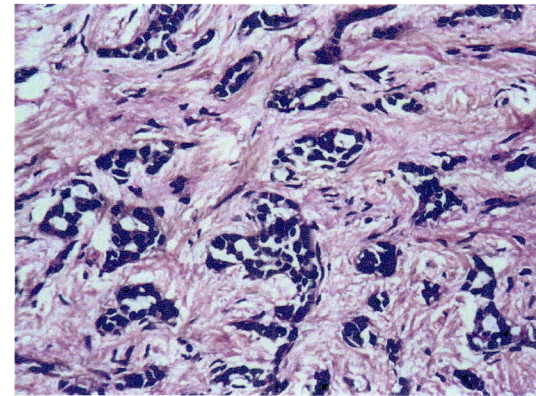

图 122 低分化胰腺癌
Poorly differentiated carcinoma of pancreas
癌细胞大部分形成腺腔，腺腔大小不一，形态不规则，肿瘤细胞异型性明显，核深染。周围有纤维结缔组织间质

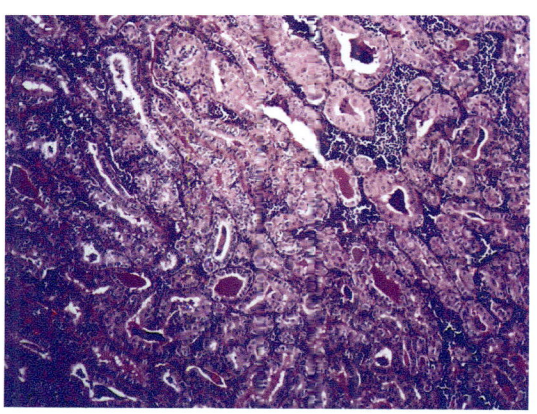

图 123 甲状腺滤泡状腺癌
（低倍镜）
Thyroid follicular adenocarcinoma
瘤细胞增生呈滤泡样结构，小部分呈实性细胞团

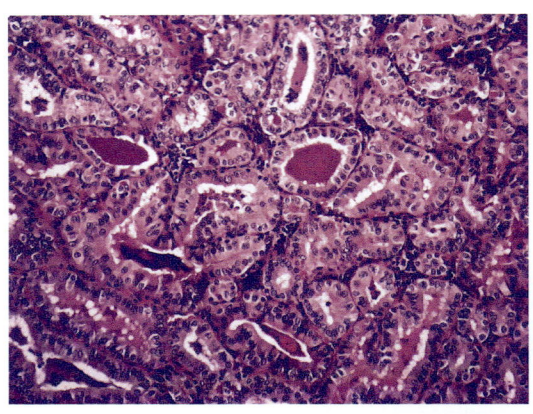

图124　甲状腺滤泡状腺癌
（高倍镜）
Thyroid follicular adenocarcinoma
瘤细胞增生呈滤泡样结构，分化程度不同，核染色质丰富

图125　甲状腺乳头状癌
Thyroid papillary carcinoma
癌细胞围绕纤维血管中心轴呈乳头状排列，分支小而多，核染色质少，呈毛玻璃状

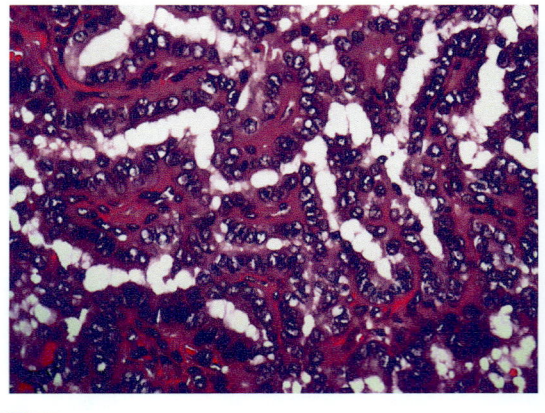

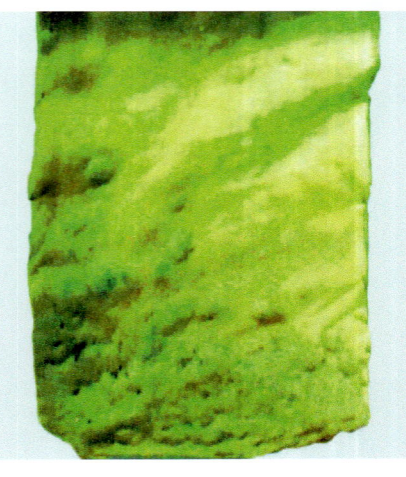

图126　肝癌腹膜种植转移
Liver carcinoma seeding to peritoneum
腹膜上可见到多个肿瘤转移结节

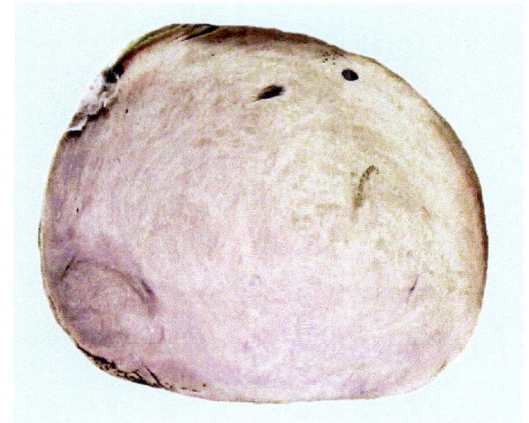

图 127 纤维瘤
Fibroma
外观呈球形肿物，与周围组织分界清楚，有包膜，切面灰白色，可见编织状或漩涡状排列的纤维条纹，质韧硬

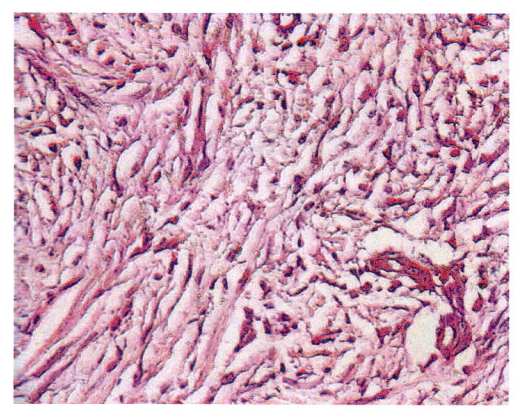

图 128 纤维瘤
Fibroma
肿瘤细胞与正常纤维细胞相似，但数量增多，且排列紊乱，纤维数目也增多

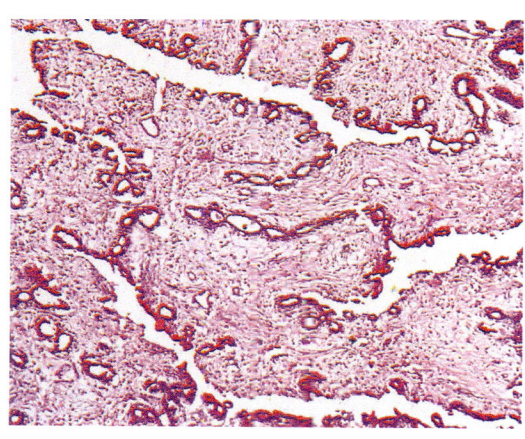

图 129 乳腺纤维腺瘤
Fibroadenama of breast
肿瘤实质成分为两种，增生的编织状排列的纤维样组织以及增生的呈腺瘤样结构的瘤组织，腺腔被挤压，不规则花边样

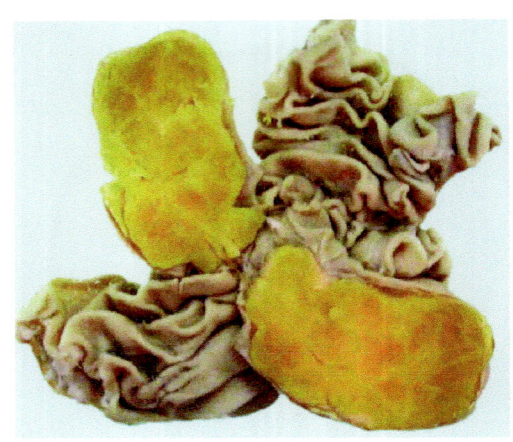

图 130　脂肪瘤
Lipoma
肠黏膜表面可见一指状肿物，表面完整，切面黄色，有完整包膜

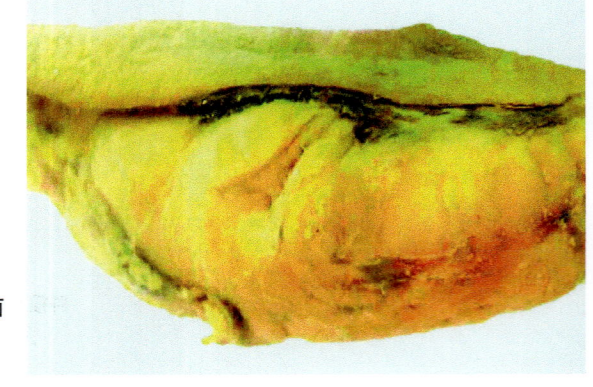

图 131　脂肪瘤
Lipoma
皮下肿瘤，有完整包膜，表面完整黄色

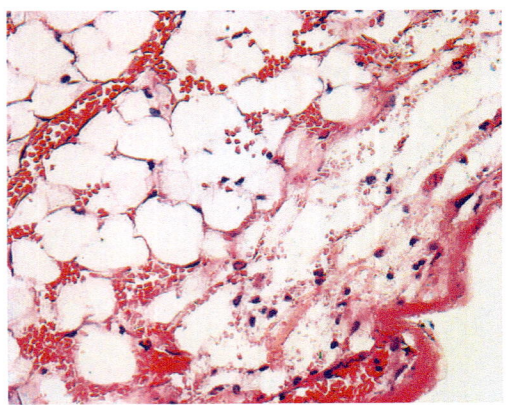

图 132　脂肪瘤
Lipoma
肿瘤有纤维性包膜，类似正常脂肪组织，呈不规则分叶状，有纤维间隔

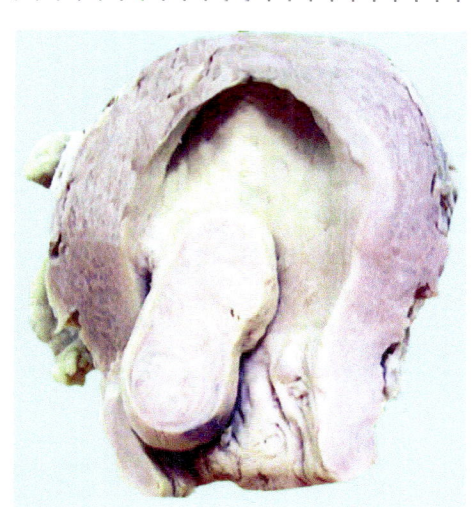

图133 子宫平滑肌瘤
Leiomyoma of uterus
肿瘤单发，位于子宫内膜下，切面呈灰红色，有包膜，切面可见编织状纹理

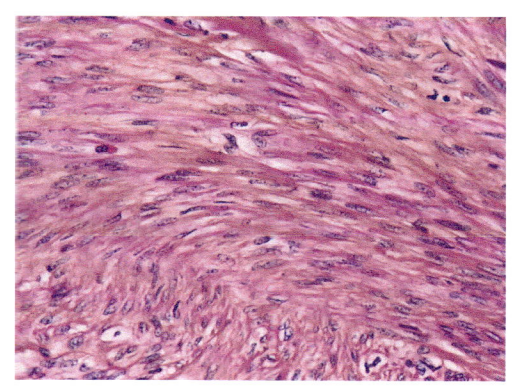

图134 子宫平滑肌瘤
Leiomyoma of uterus
肿瘤组织由形态比较一致的梭形平滑肌细胞构成。细胞排列成束，互相编织，核呈长杆状，两端钝圆

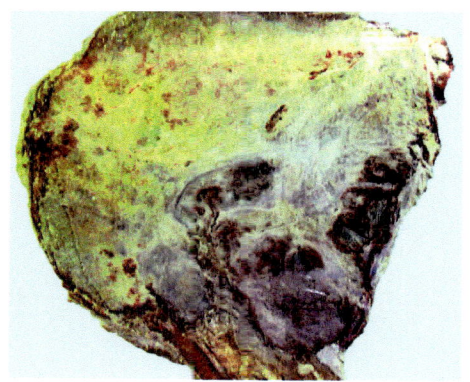

图135 骨肉瘤
Osteosarcoma
长骨末端可见一肿物，质硬，切面肿瘤呈多彩样变化，其中成骨多处呈现黄白色，成骨少处呈灰红色，部分出血呈红褐色

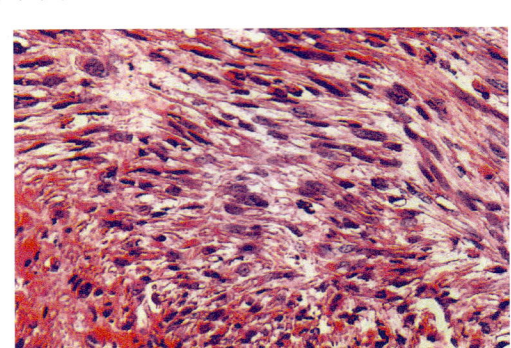

图136　纤维肉瘤
Fibrosarcoma
肿瘤细胞异型性明显，核椭圆形或梭形，偶见瘤巨细胞，肿瘤实质、间质交错存在，纤维成分较少，部分区域黏液变性明显，瘤细胞呈星形或多边形

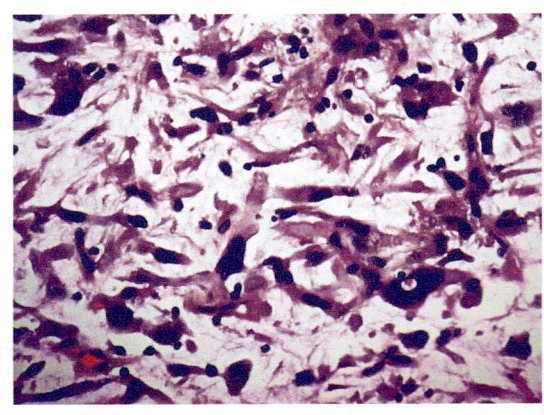

图137　横纹肌肉瘤
Rhabdomyosarcoma
肉瘤细胞呈散在分布，细胞胞浆宽广，部分细胞保留横纹肌细胞胞体柱状分化的形态特点。瘤细胞核浓染，核与细胞均呈多态性，可见瘤巨细胞

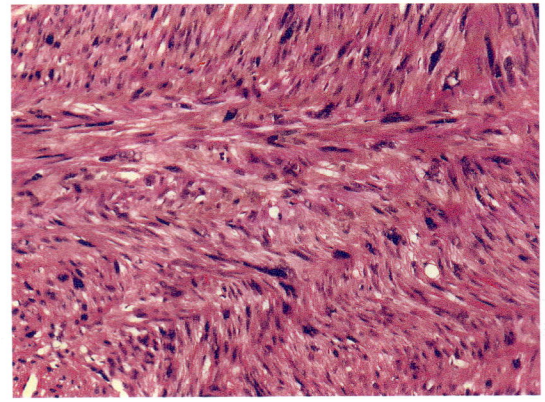

图138　平滑肌肉瘤（低倍镜）
Leiomyosarcoma
肿瘤细胞分化不成熟，排列呈束状、编织状。瘤细胞丰富而拥挤，且细胞膜界限不清，使胞核明显密集，核的异型性明显

第1篇 病理学总论

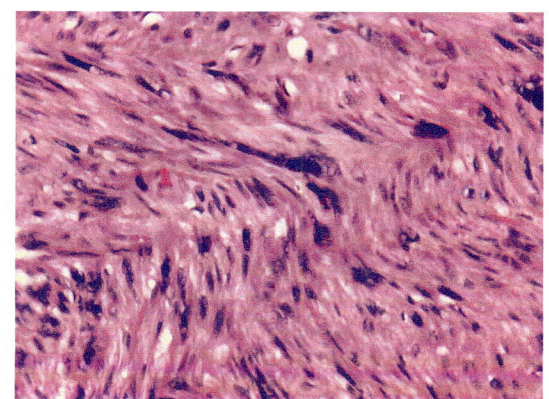

图139 平滑肌肉瘤（高倍镜）
Leiomyosarcoma
瘤细胞异型性明显，细胞核浓染，核大小不等，长短不一，呈不规则带状、杆状和梭形，多处可见瘤巨细胞

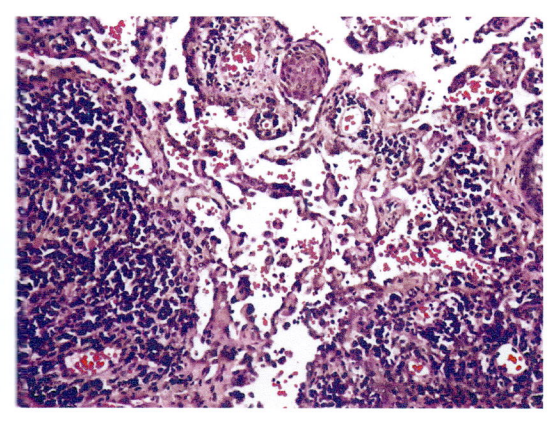

图140 皮肤血管肉瘤
Hemangiosarcoma of skin
肉瘤细胞形成血管样结构，也可聚集成片状，瘤细胞异型性明显

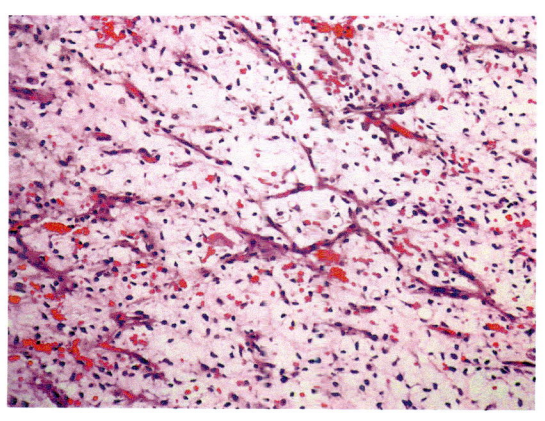

图141 脂肪肉瘤
Liposarcoma
瘤组织可见散在脂肪母细胞，胞体较大，胞浆内含有多少不等的脂滴。制片后溶解形成脂肪空泡，同时可见血管呈枝丫状分布

47

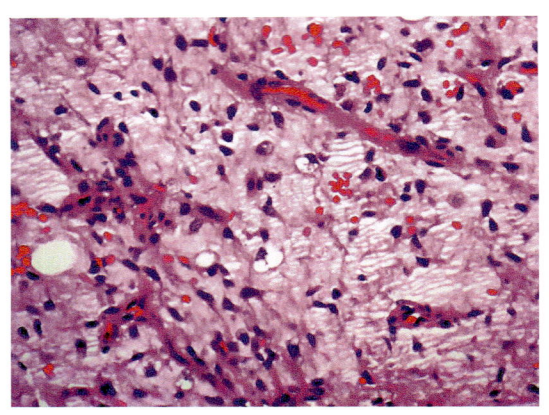

图 142　脂肪肉瘤
Liposarcoma
高倍镜显示脂肪母细胞核呈三角形、梭形或多变形，细胞内的脂滴将胞核挤向一侧，脂肪母细胞一般较正常脂肪细胞小，且具有明显异型性，是脂肪肉瘤的重要特点，有利于诊断

图 143　混合痣（低倍镜）
Junctional nevus
痣细胞见于表皮和真皮内，可见从表皮"滴落"到真皮内

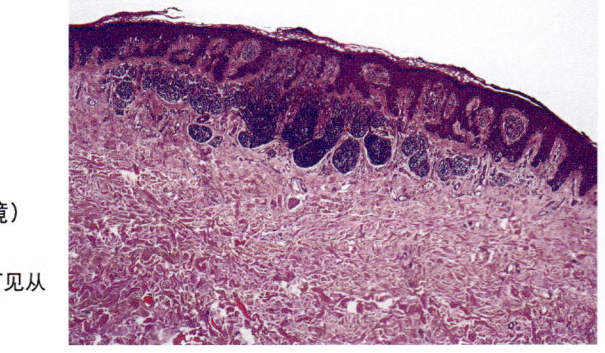

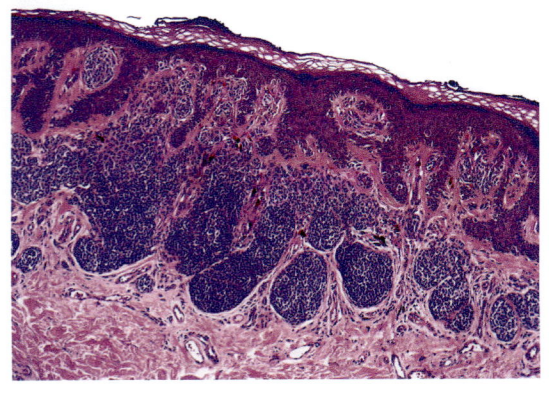

图 144　混合痣（高倍镜）
Junctional nevus
痣细胞见于表皮和真皮内，可见从表皮"滴落"到真皮内

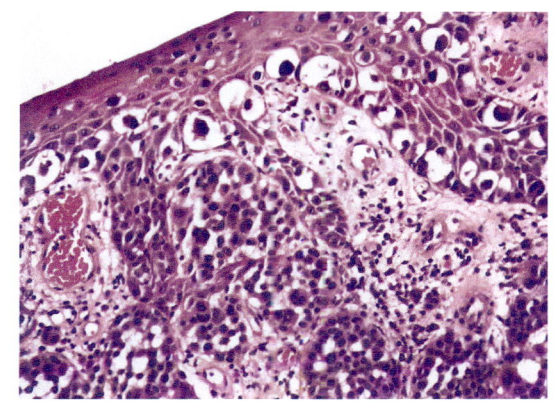

图 145 背部黑色素瘤
Melanoma of back
表皮基底层破坏,瘤细胞浸润到真皮乳头层和网状层

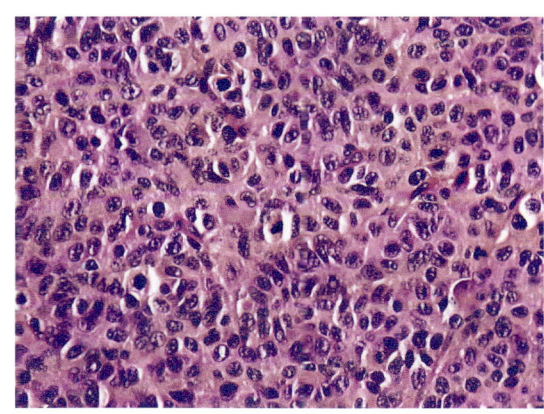

图 146 背部黑色素瘤
Melanoma of back
瘤细胞大,排列呈巢或腺泡状。异型性大,有多个病理性核分裂象

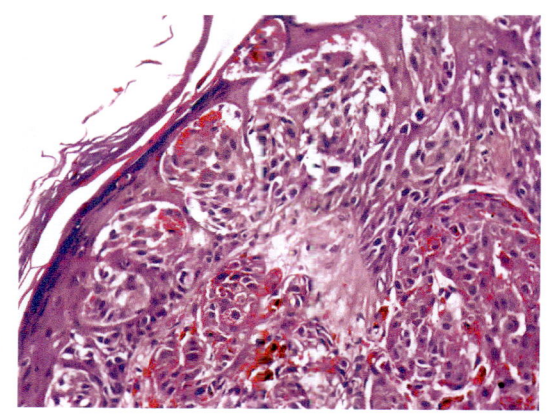

图 147 前臂痣恶变的黑色素瘤
Melanoma from nevus of forearm
真皮内和网状层有许多瘤细胞,细胞多为梭形,有异型性。黑色素多

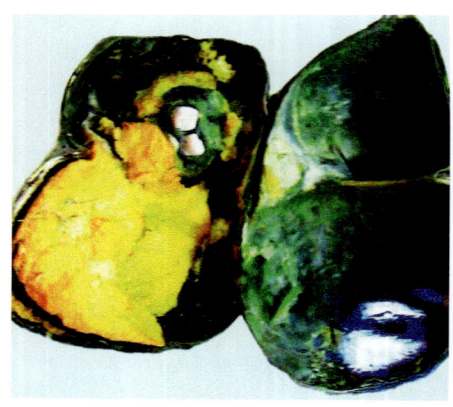

图148 卵巢囊性成熟性畸胎瘤
Mature cystic teratoma of ovary
肿瘤表面光滑，切开为囊性，囊腔内充满黄色脂质，少量毛发和牙齿

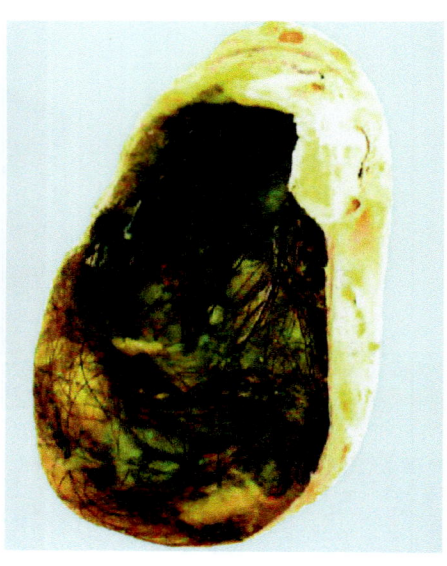

图149 卵巢囊性成熟性畸胎瘤
Mature cystic teratoma of ovary
肿瘤表面光滑，切开为囊性，囊腔内充满毛发和黄色脂质

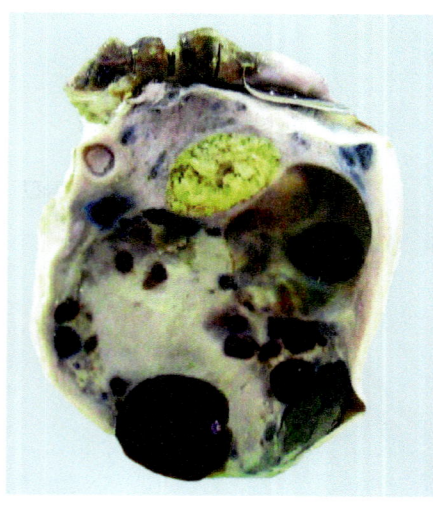

图150 卵巢实性成熟性畸胎瘤
Mature solid teratoma of ovary
肿瘤表面光滑，界限清楚，切开为灰红色实性肿物，并可见黑（红）色肾上腺，褐色甲状腺及黄色脂质

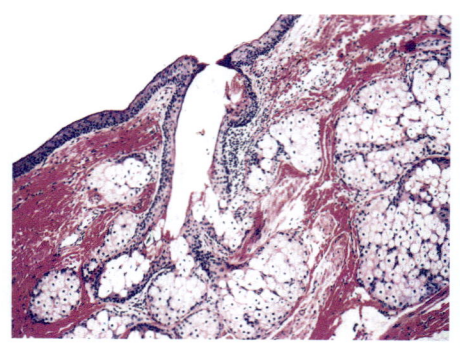

图151 卵巢成熟性畸胎瘤
Mature teratoma of ovary
卵巢肿瘤组织为分化成熟的皮肤组织：表皮、毛囊、皮脂腺及竖毛肌

病理学各论
SYSTEMIC PATHOLOGY

第 2 篇

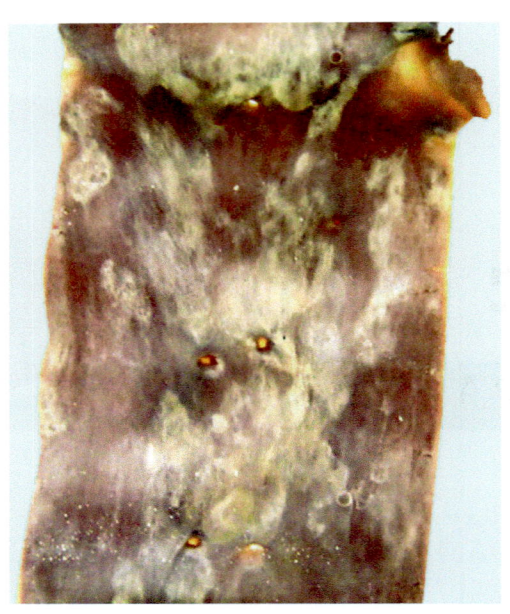

图152 纤维斑块
Fibrous plaque
剖开之胸主动脉可见散在不规则
隆起的斑块，呈瓷白色

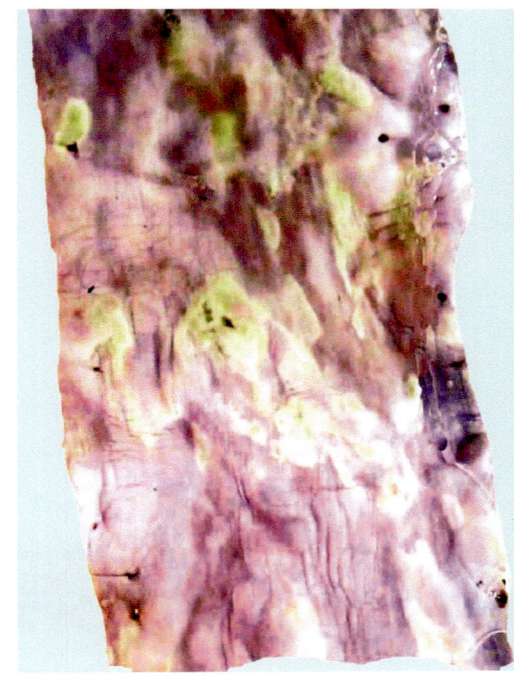

图153 粥样斑块
Atheromatous plaque
剖开之胸主动脉可见灰黄色斑块明显
隆起于内膜表面

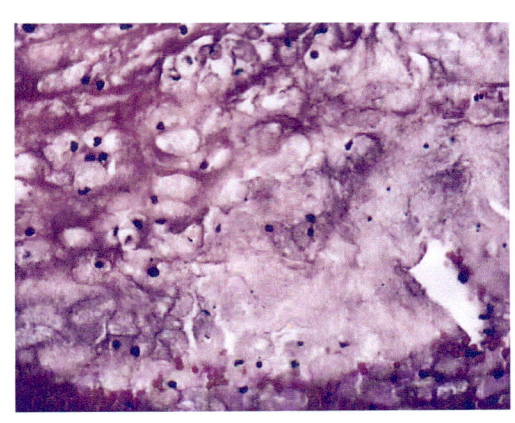

图 154 脂纹
Fatty streak
大量泡沫细胞堆集于内膜层,泡沫细胞体积大,圆形,胞浆内有大量小空泡

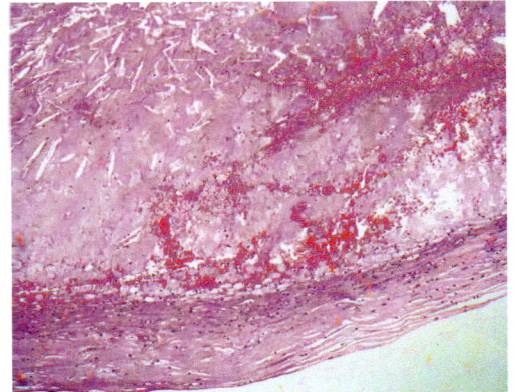

图 155 粥样斑块
Atheromatous plaque
表层为纤维帽,深部为大量不定形坏死崩解产物、胆固醇结晶、泡沫细胞和少量淋巴细胞

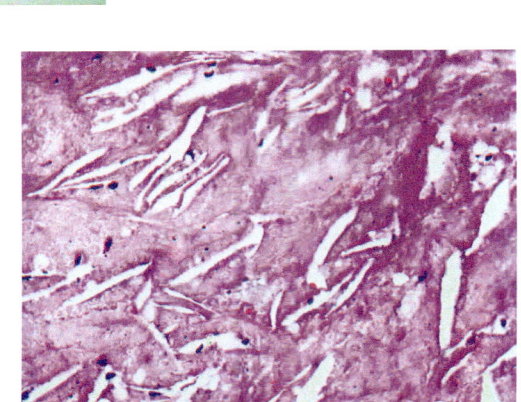

图 156 粥样斑块
Atheromatous plaque
胆固醇结晶呈针状空隙

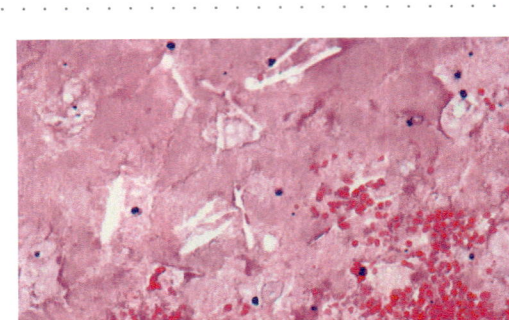

图 157 斑块内出血
Hemorrhage in atheromatous plaque
斑块内新生的血管破裂，红细胞漏出

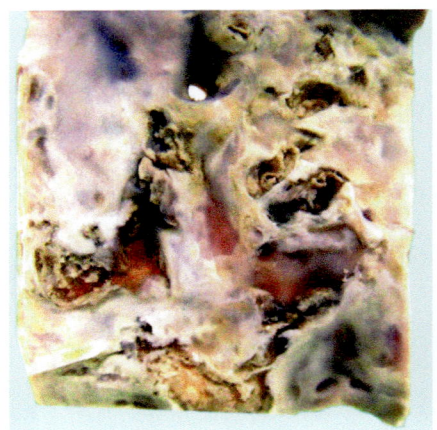

图 158 斑块破裂
Cracking of atheromatous plaque
斑块表面的纤维帽破裂，遗留粥瘤样溃疡

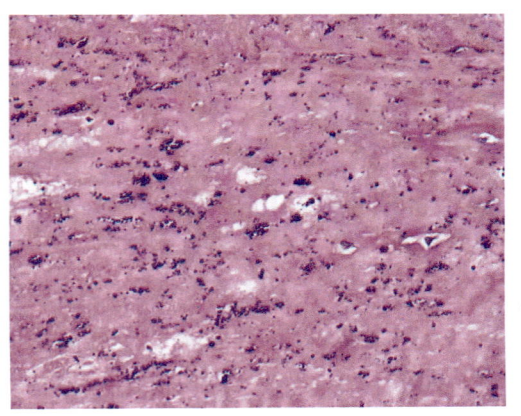

图 159 斑块钙化
Calcification of atheromatous plaque
纤维帽和粥瘤病灶内可见蓝色颗粒状钙盐沉积

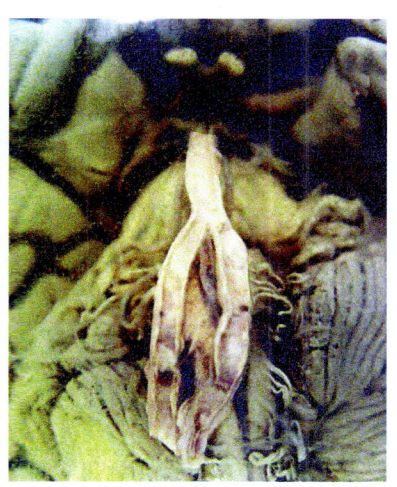

图 160 脑动脉粥样硬化
Cerebral artery atherosclerosis
剖开之脑基底动脉内可见粥样斑块

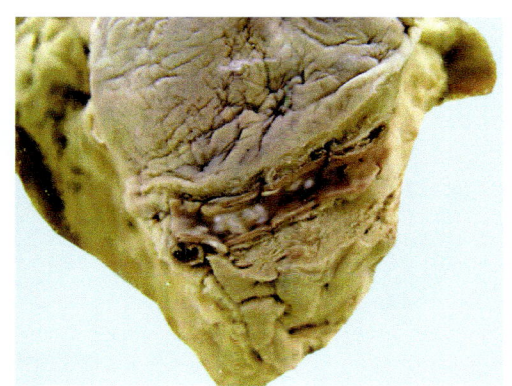

图 161 冠状动脉粥样硬化
Coronary atherosclerosis
剖开之冠状动脉内可见粥样斑块

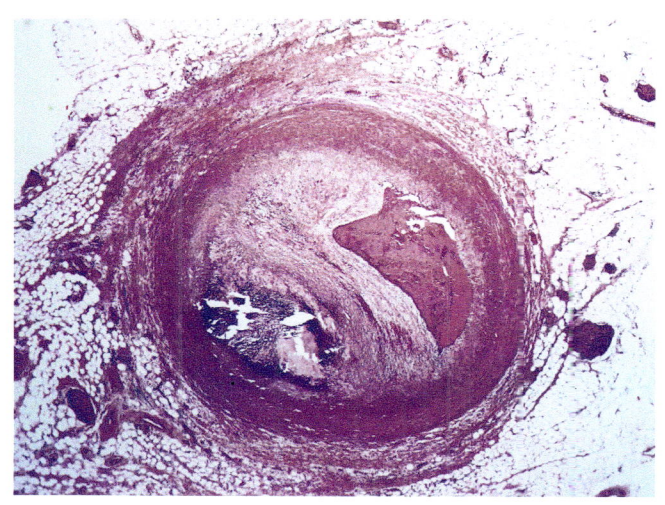

图 162 冠状动脉粥样硬化
Coronary atherosclerosis
冠状动脉内可见粥样斑块呈新月状，有钙盐沉积

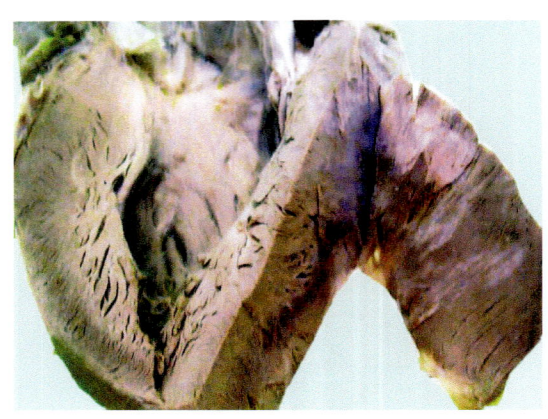

图163　陈旧性心肌梗死
Stale myocardial infarction
病灶心肌呈灰白色条索状

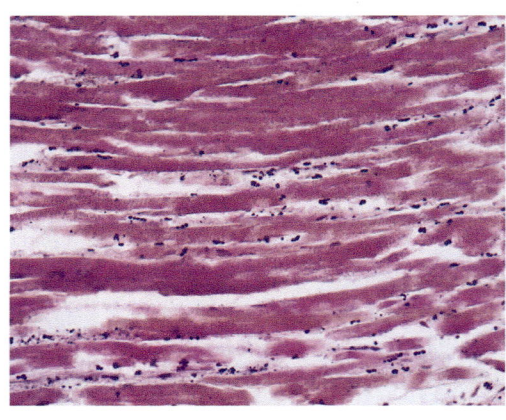

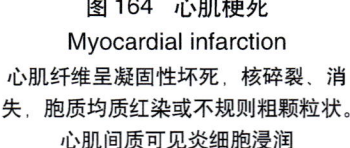

图164　心肌梗死
Myocardial infarction
心肌纤维呈凝固性坏死，核碎裂、消失，胞质均质红染或不规则粗颗粒状。心肌间质可见炎细胞浸润

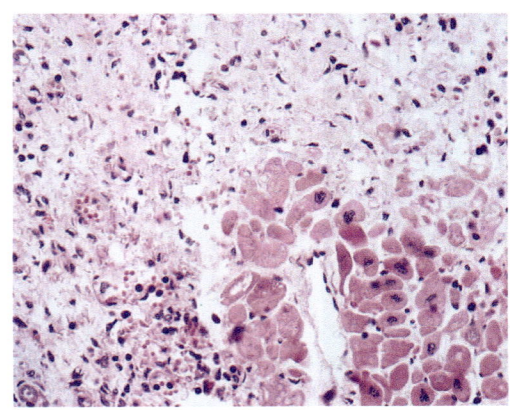

图165　心肌梗死
Myocardial infarction
梗死灶被肉芽组织取代

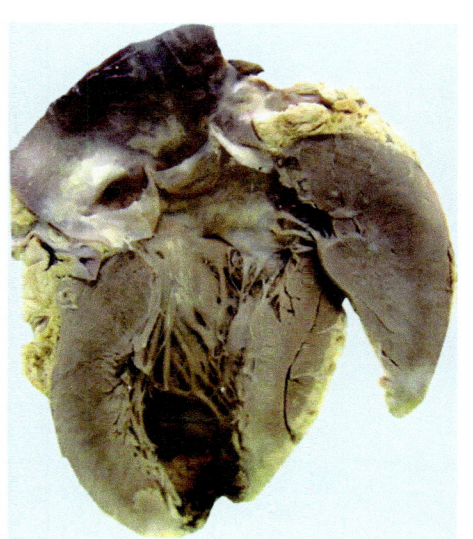

图 166 心脏破裂
Rupture of heart
心尖处可见陈旧瘢痕、室壁瘤及心室壁破裂

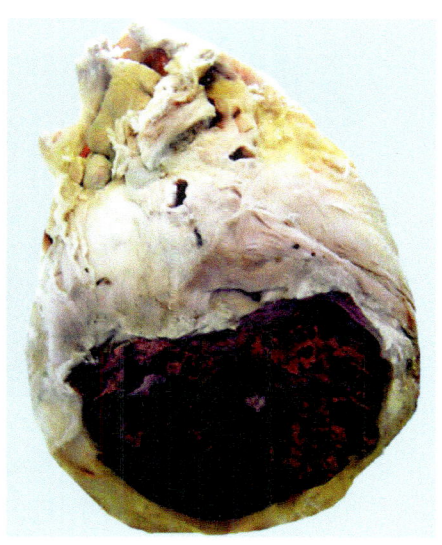

图 167 心包填塞
Tamponade in pericardium
心脏破裂后血液溢入心包腔造成急性心包填塞

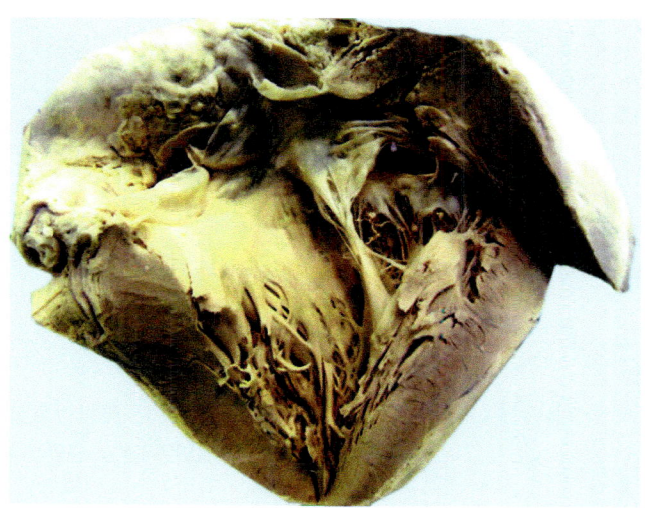

图 168 高血压心脏病合并主动脉粥样硬化
Hypertensive heart disease with aorta atherosclerosis
左心室壁增厚，乳头肌和肉柱增粗，主动脉开口处有黄色粥样斑块

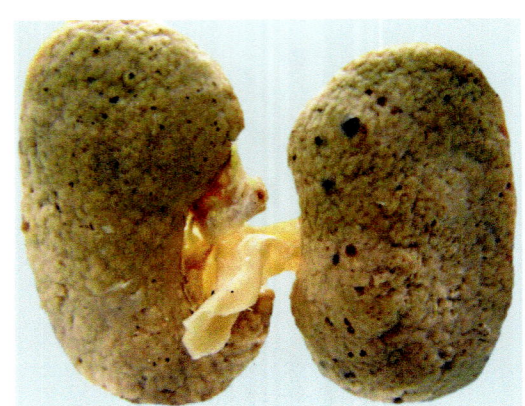

图169 原发性颗粒性固缩肾
Primary granular atrophy of kidney
双侧肾脏对称性缩小，重量减轻，质地变硬，表面呈均匀弥漫的细颗粒状

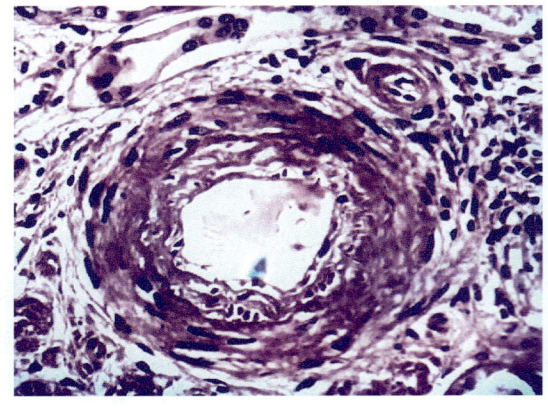

图170 原发性颗粒性固缩肾
Primary granular atrophy of kidney
肌型小动脉内膜胶原纤维及弹性纤维增生，中膜平滑肌细胞增生，管壁增厚，管腔狭窄

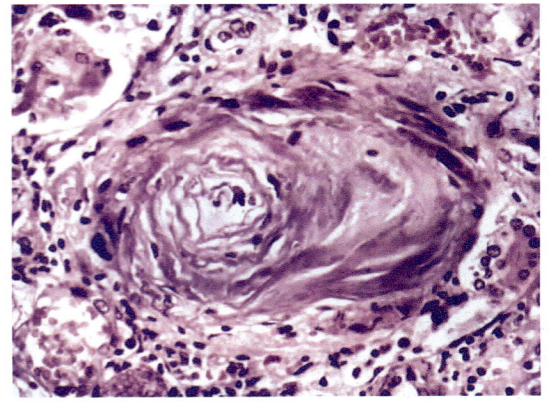

图171 原发性颗粒性固缩肾
Primary granular atrophy of kidney
肌型小动脉内膜胶原纤维及弹性纤维增生，中膜平滑肌细胞增生，管壁增厚，管腔狭窄

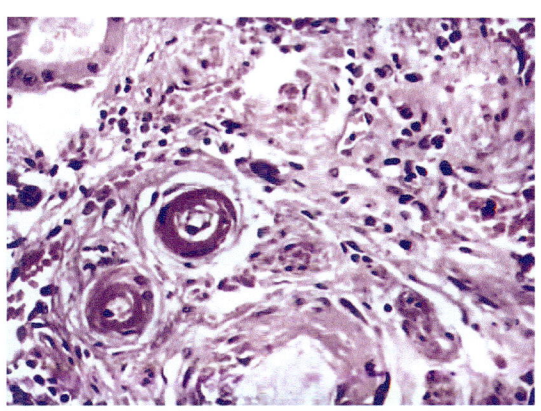

图 172　原发性颗粒性固缩肾
Primary granular atrophy of kidney
入球小动脉内膜下可见均质红染无结构玻璃样物质，导致管壁增厚　管腔缩小

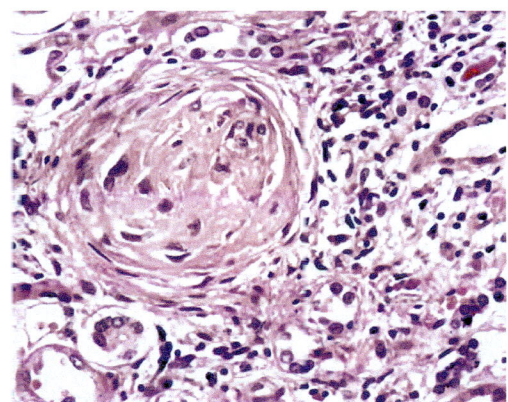

图 173　原发性颗粒性固缩肾
Primary granular atrophy of kidney
病变区肾小球缺血发生纤维化和玻璃样变性

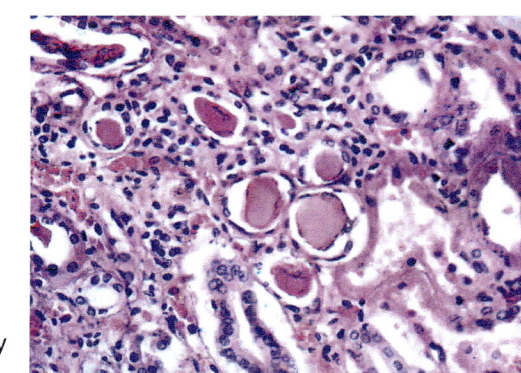

图 174　原发性颗粒性固缩肾
Primary granular atrophy of kidney
病变区肾小管内可见蛋白管型

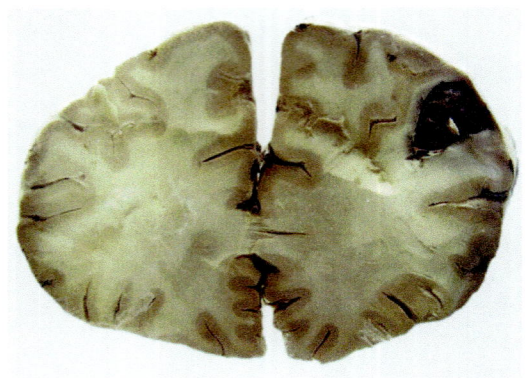

图175　脑出血
Haemorrhage in cerebra
出血部位脑组织完全破坏，形成充满血液和坏死脑组织的囊性病灶

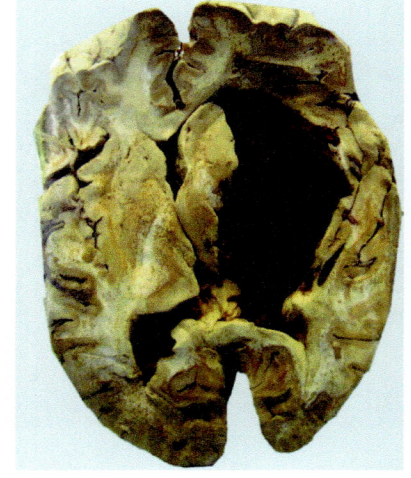

图176　脑出血
Haemorrhage in cerebra
出血量大，破入脑室内，形成充满血液和坏死脑组织的囊性病灶

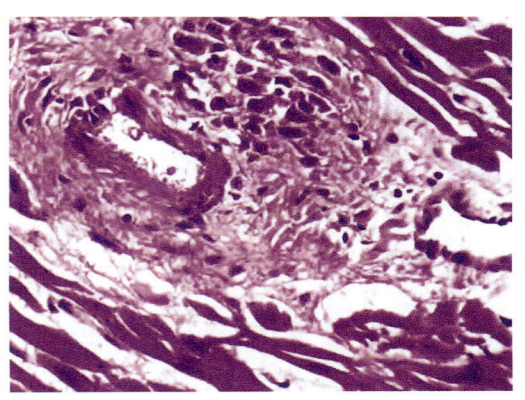

图177　风湿小结
Aschoff body
中心为纤维素样坏死，周边为成团的风湿细胞，伴有淋巴细胞、浆细胞

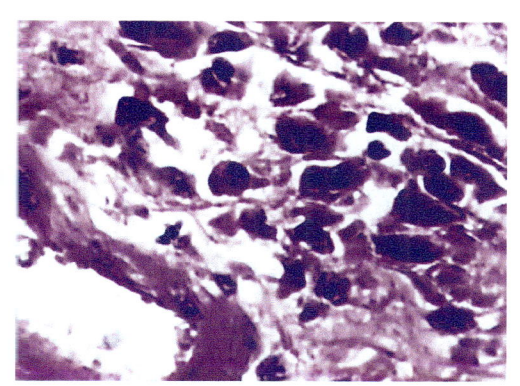

图 178　风湿细胞
Aschoff cell
风湿细胞体积大，圆形，胞质丰富，核大，圆形或椭圆形，核膜清楚，染色质集中于中央，横切面似枭眼样，纵切面呈毛虫样

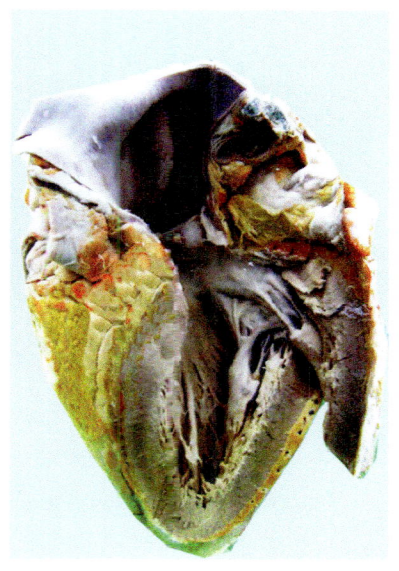

图 179　风湿性心内膜炎
Rheumatic endocarditis
瓣膜闭锁缘上形成疣状赘生物，灰白色半透明，附着牢固，不易脱落

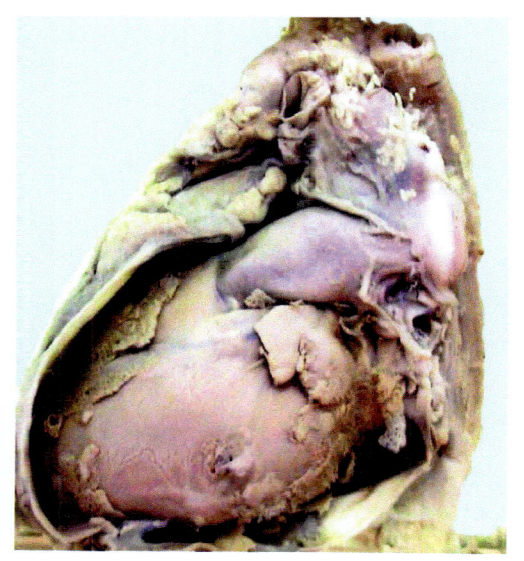

图 180　风湿性心外膜炎
Rheumatic pericarditis
覆盖于心外膜表面的纤维素形成绒毛状外观

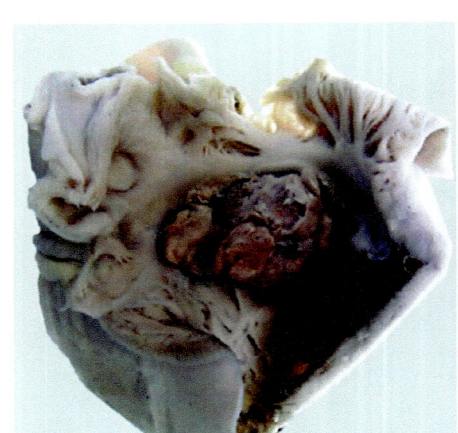

图181 急性感染性心内膜炎
Acute infective endocarditis
心瓣膜上可见疣状赘生物,体积庞大,灰黄色,瓣膜完全被破坏

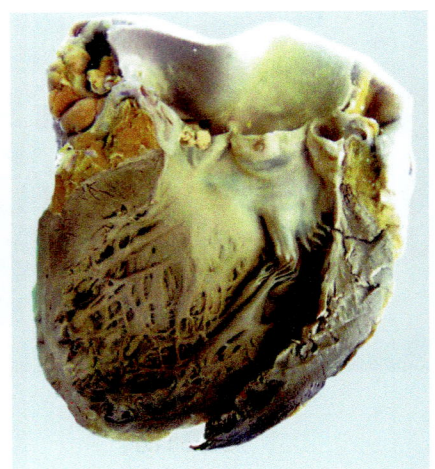

图182 亚急性感染性心内膜炎
Subacute infective endocarditis
心瓣膜上可见疣状赘生物,呈小菜花状,质松脆,易破碎、脱落

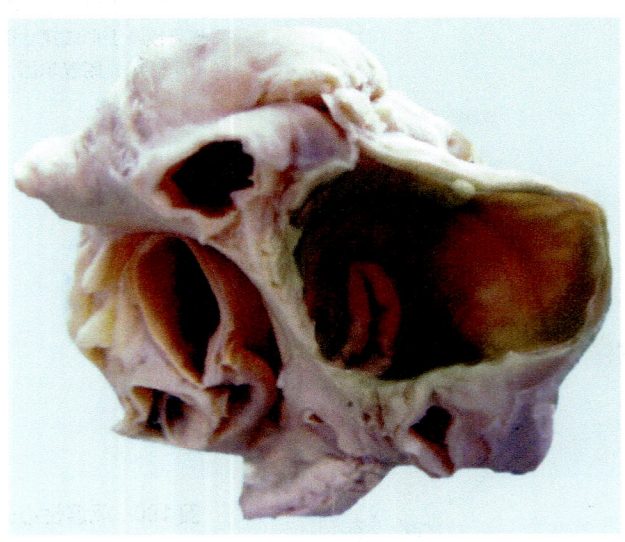

图183 慢性瓣膜病
Chronic valvular vitium of heart
二尖瓣瓣膜增厚、变硬、粘连,腱索缩短,瓣膜呈鱼口状

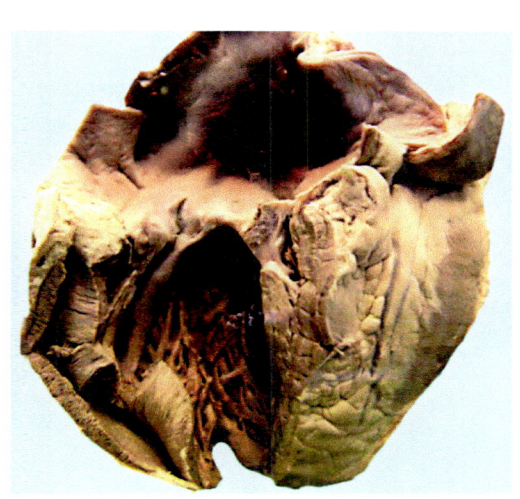

图 184 慢性瓣膜病
Chronic valvular vitium of heart
瓣膜增厚、变硬、卷曲、缩短、粘连

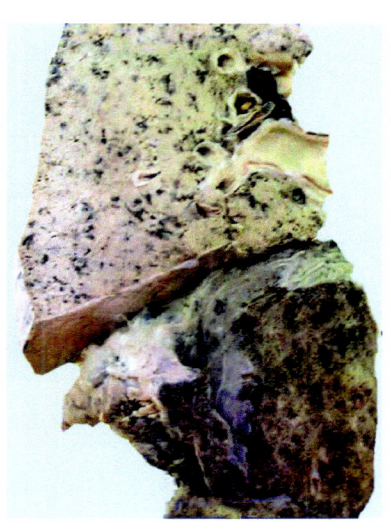

图 185 大叶性肺炎（灰色肝样变期）
Lobar pneumonia (stage of gray hepatization)
左肺上叶为病变区域，色灰白，干燥，质实似肝，切面呈细颗粒状。下叶可见代偿性肺气肿

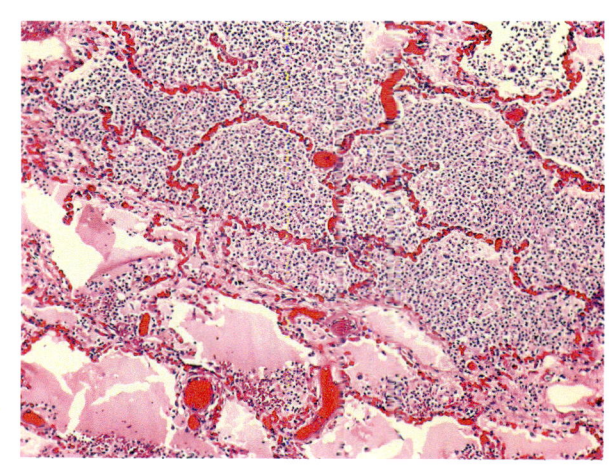

图 186 大叶性肺炎（灰色肝样变早期）
Lobar pneumonia (early stage of gray hepatization)
肺泡壁毛细血管轻度扩张充血，肺泡腔内大量纤维素渗出，部分肺泡腔内可见水肿液

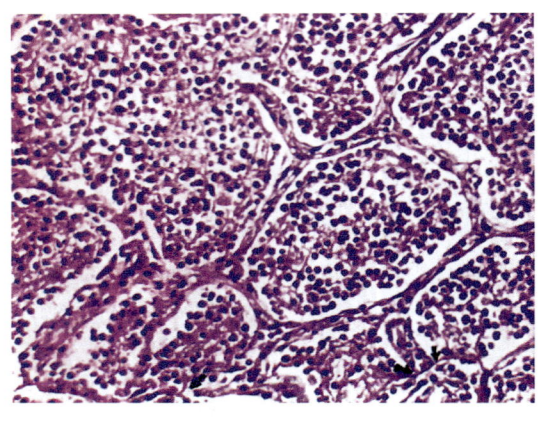

图187 大叶性肺炎（灰色肝样变早期）
Lobar pneumonia (stage of gray hepatization)
肺泡壁完好，肺泡腔内有大量纤维素渗出，相互交织成网状，网眼中可见大量中性粒细胞浸润，相邻肺泡腔内纤维素通过肺泡间孔彼此相连

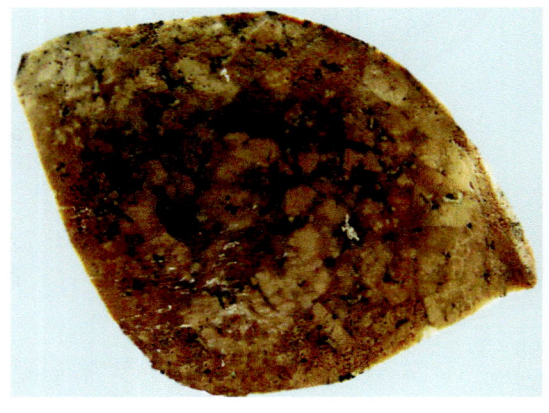

图188 小叶性肺炎
Lobular pneumonia
病变呈灶状分布，病灶大小不一，形态不规则，部分有融合。病灶中央可见病变细支气管横断面

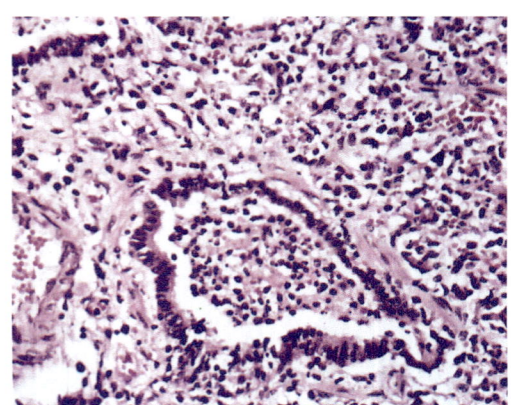

图189 小叶性肺炎
Lobular pneumonia
中央为病变细支气管，管腔内及其周围肺组织内可见以中性粒细胞为主的炎性渗出物

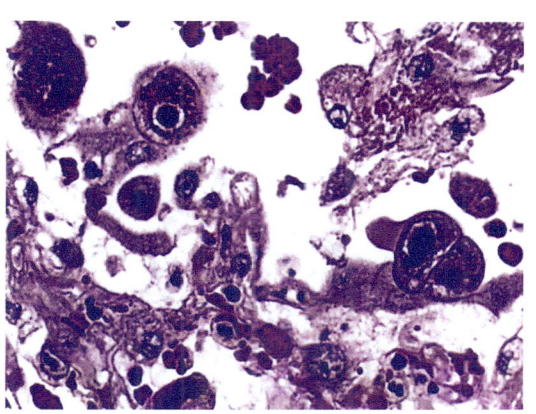

图 190 病毒性肺炎（病毒包涵体）
Viral pneumonia (viral inclusion bodies)
肺泡上皮细胞核内可见病毒包涵体，呈圆形或椭圆形，约为红细胞大小，周围有清晰的透明晕

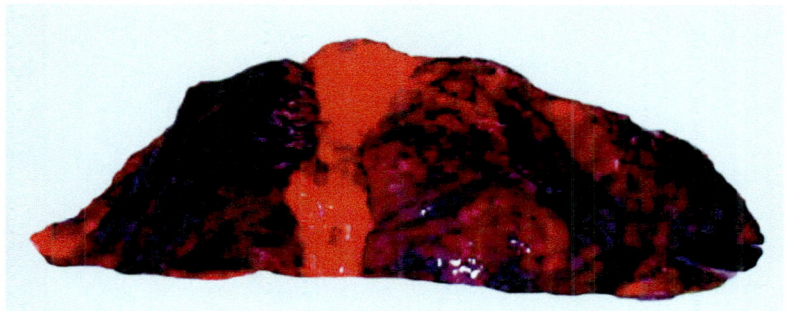

图 191 严重急性呼吸综合征（SARS）
Severe acute respiratory syndrome
肺组织明显膨胀，充血出血，表面暗红色，质实

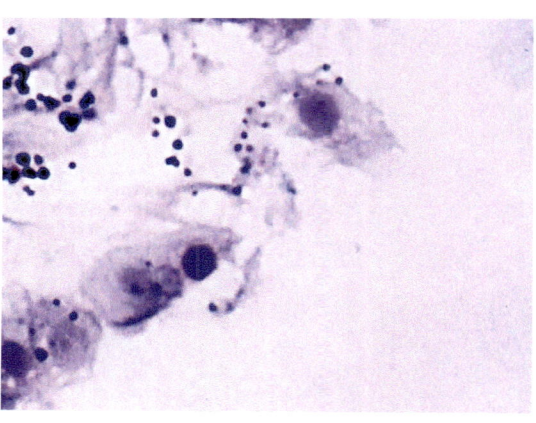

图 192 严重急性呼吸综合征（SARS）
Severe acute respiratory syndrome
肺泡上皮细胞质内可见紫蓝色的病毒颗粒，形成球形病毒包涵体，与胞浆之间有透明晕相隔

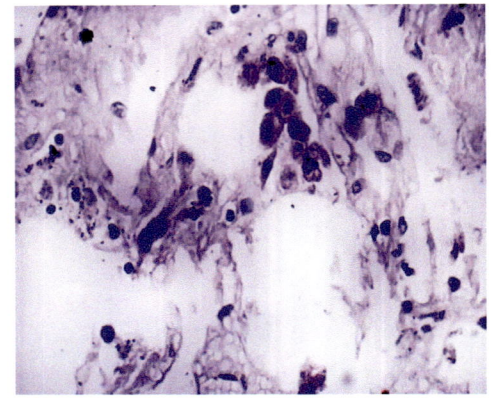

图193 严重急性呼吸综合征（SARS）
Severe acute respiratory syndrome
免疫组织化学染色显示胞浆内冠状病毒蛋白
（SARS-CoV）

图194 严重急性呼吸综合征
（SARS）
Severe acute respiratory
syndrome
肺泡腔内见浆液性渗出物，部分渗出物沿肺泡腔面浓缩形成均质红染膜样物，即透明膜

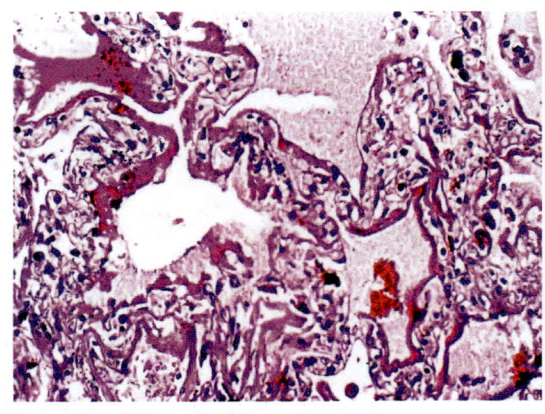

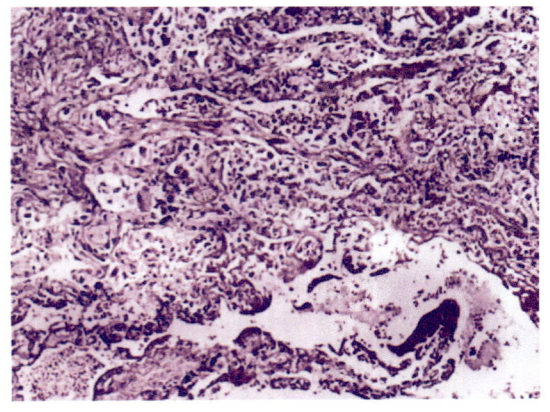

图195 严重急性呼吸综合征
（SARS）
Severe acute respiratory
syndrome
肺组织内见弥漫性纤维组织增生，部分呈机化性肺炎改变

图 196 严重急性呼吸综合征（SARS）（肺门淋巴结）
Severe acute respiratory syndrome (lymph node at hilum of lung)
淋巴结结构消失，小血管扩张充血。淋巴细胞数量明显减少。被膜下窦内有较多单核细胞浸润

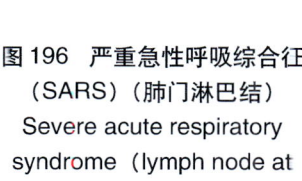
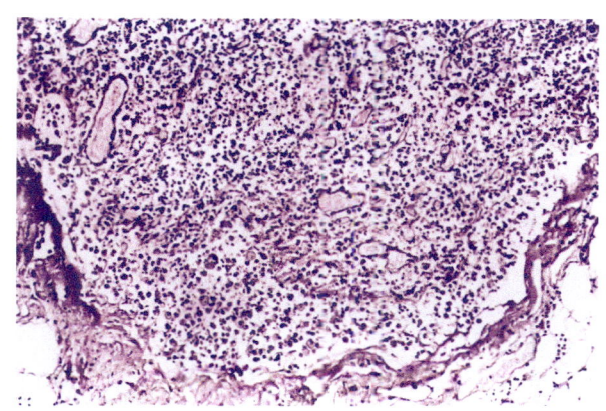

图 197 严重急性呼吸综合征（SARS）伴曲菌感染
Severe acute respiratory syndrome with aspergillus infection
肺组织中见放射状排列的黑色曲菌菌丝，菌丝较细，分支呈锐角（六胺银染色）

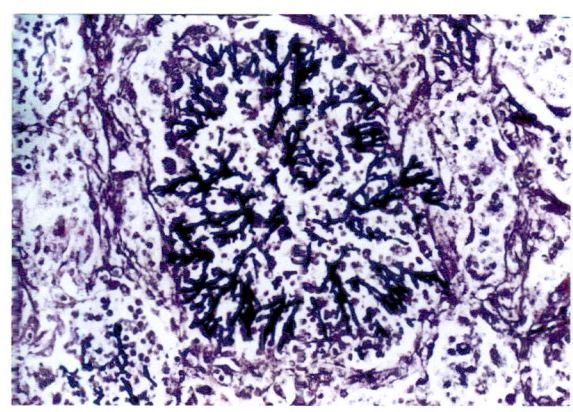

图 198 支气管哮喘
Bronchial asthma
支气管黏膜上皮增生，杯状细胞增多，上皮呈乳头状向管腔内突入。基底膜增厚并有玻璃样变。管壁平滑肌增生明显。管腔内可见黏液栓

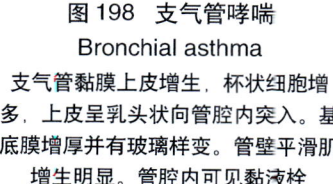
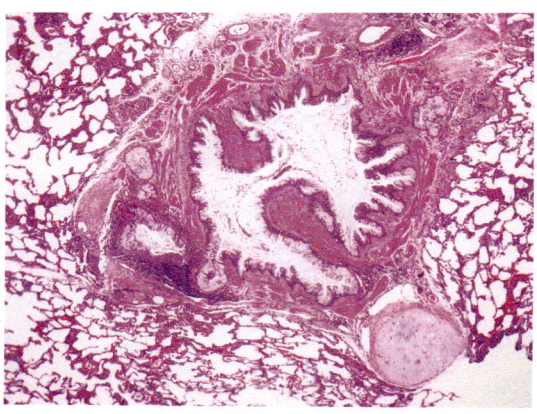

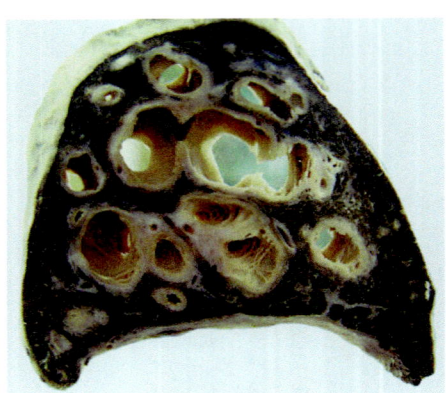

图 199 支气管扩张症
Bronchiectasis
肺组织切面可见多个明显扩张的支气管

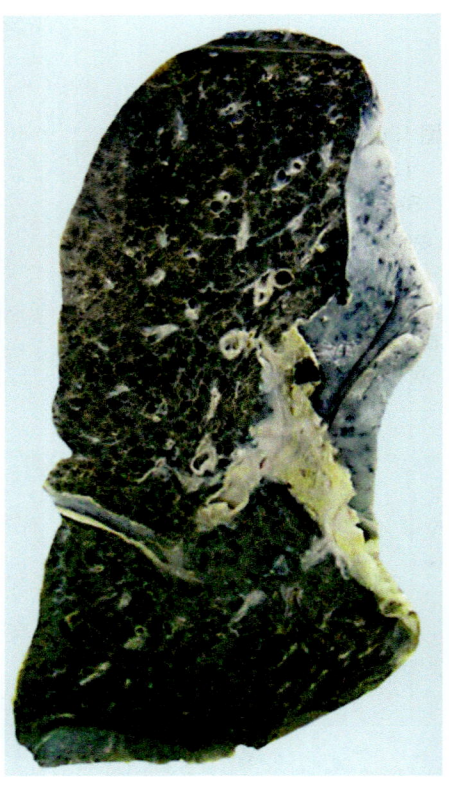

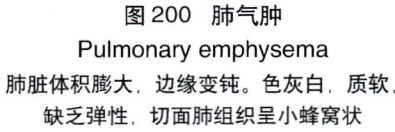

图 200 肺气肿
Pulmonary emphysema
肺脏体积膨大，边缘变钝。色灰白，质软，缺乏弹性，切面肺组织呈小蜂窝状

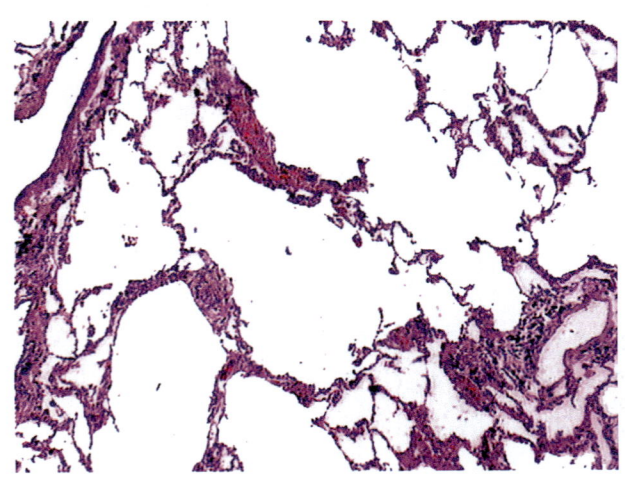

图 201 肺气肿
Pulmonary emphysema
肺泡间隔破坏，相邻肺泡融合为较大的囊腔

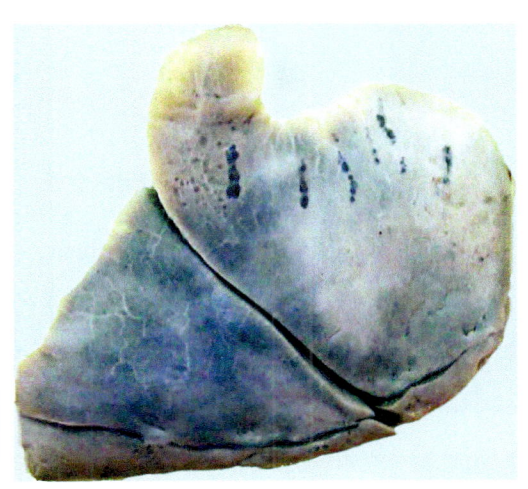

图 202　间质性肺气肿
Interstitial emphysema
图为小儿肺脏。于肺上叶边缘邻近肺膜处，可见串珠样气泡

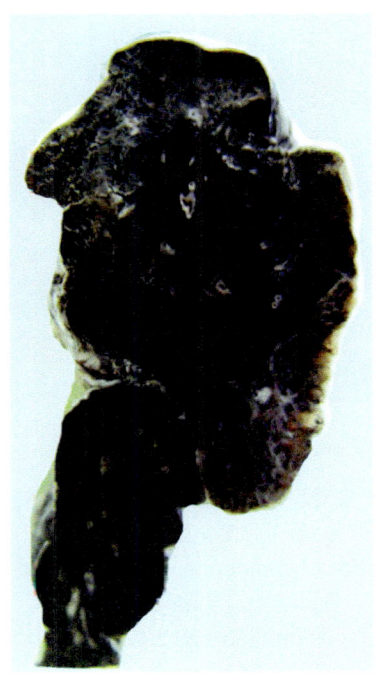

图 203　硅肺
Silicosis
肺脏体积缩小，质硬，部分实变，并可见代偿性肺气肿，局部胸膜轻度纤维化

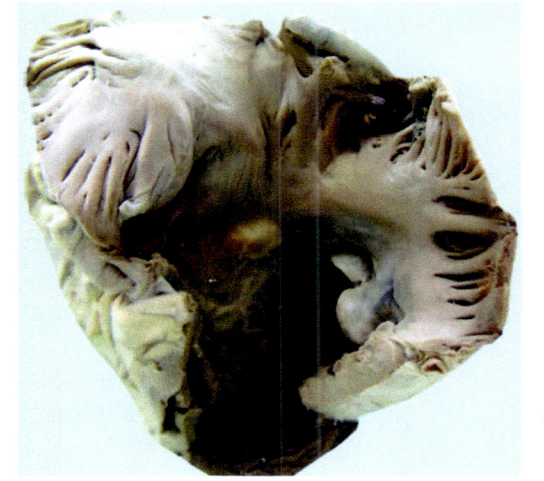

图 204　肺心病
Cor pulmonale
心脏体积增大，右室壁增厚，乳头肌、肉柱增粗，右心室扩张

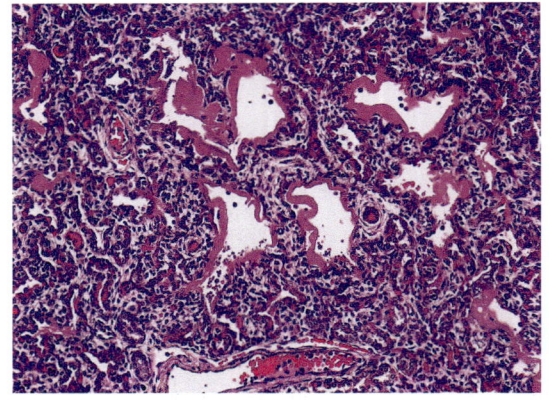

图205 新生儿呼吸窘迫综合征（NRDS）
Neonatal respiratory distress syndrome
均质红染透明膜黏附于肺泡及呼吸性细支气管内壁。肺组织大部呈肺不张状态

图206 颈淋巴结转移性鼻咽癌（非角化型鳞癌）
Neck lymph node with metastatic nasopharyngeal carcinoma (nonkeratinizing squamous cell carcinoma)
淋巴组织中见巢片状癌组织浸润。癌巢内细胞分层不明显，细胞大小不一，多呈卵圆形或梭形。肿瘤细胞间无间桥，也无角化珠形成

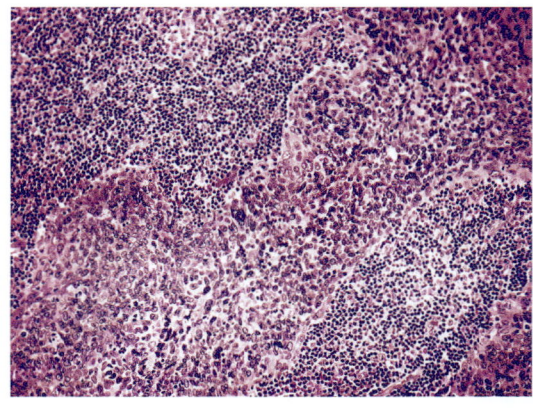

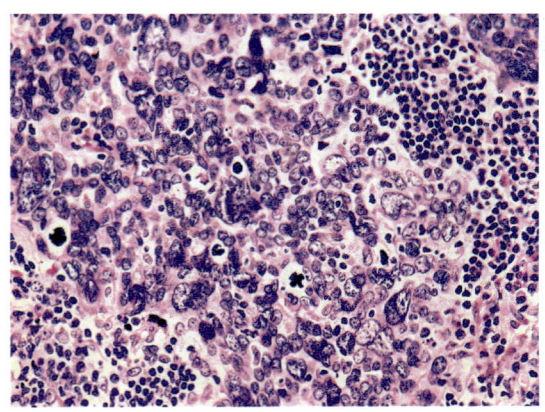

图207 颈淋巴结转移性鼻咽癌（非角化型鳞癌）
Neck lymph node with metastatic nasopharyngeal carcinoma (nonkeratinizing squamous cell carcinoma)
图206高倍图。显示癌巢内细胞及其核的多形性，并可见多个病理性核分裂象

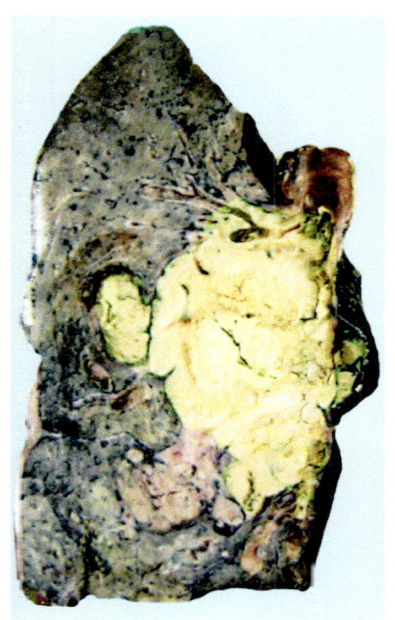

图 208 中央型肺癌
Carcinoma of lung, central type
肺门处可见包绕支气管的灰白、质硬的巨大肿块，切面灰白、质硬、干燥

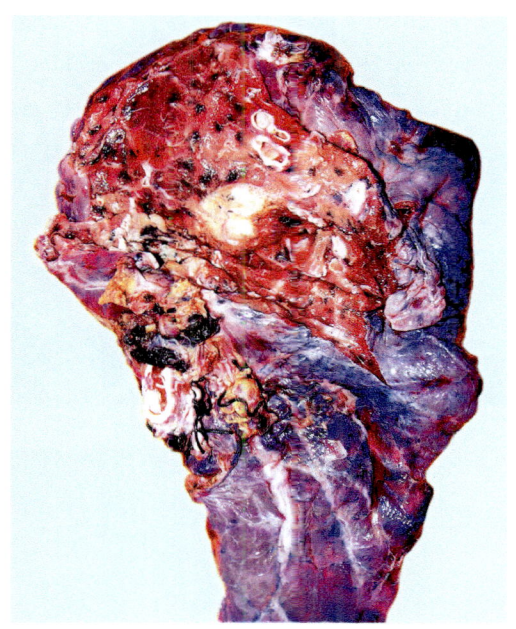

图 209 周围型肺癌
Carcinoma of lung, peripheral type
肺组织切面可见灰白色肿物，近胸膜。与周围支气管无明显关系

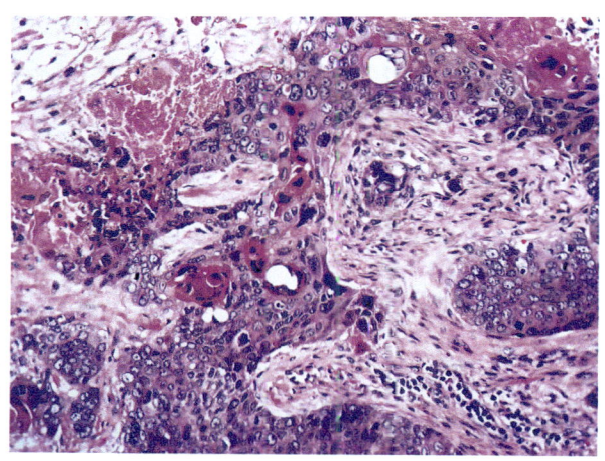

图 210 肺鳞癌
Squamous cell carcinoma of lung
癌细胞排列呈不规则巢状，癌巢内见角化。肿瘤实质与间质境界清楚

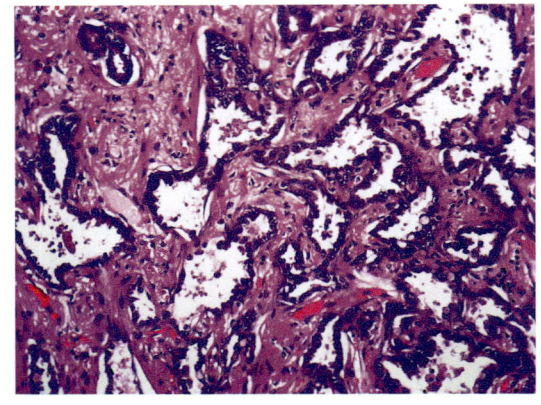

图211 肺腺癌（混合细胞型）
Adenocarcinoma of lung（mixed cell subtype）
癌细胞排列成腺腔样结构，细胞形态多样，部分为扁平，部分为立方或柱状

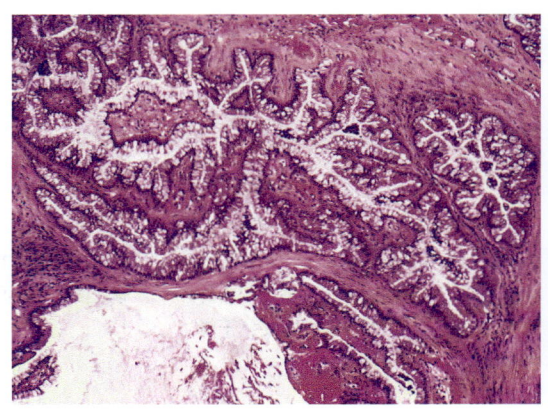

图212 肺腺癌（杯状细胞型）
Adenocarcinoma of lung（goblet cell subtype）
癌细胞排列成腺腔样结构，并有乳头状突起，部分腺腔内有黏液积聚。癌细胞异型性较小，核位于基底，似杯状细胞

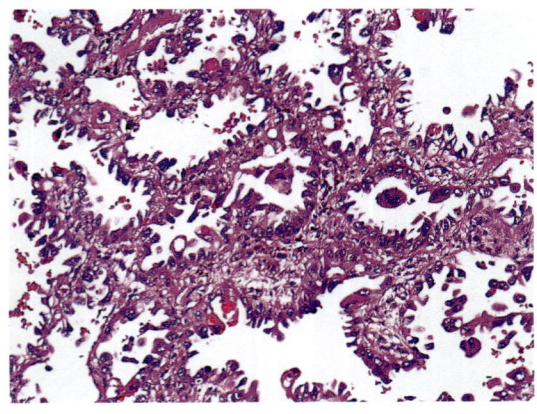

图213 肺腺癌（细支气管肺泡癌）
Adenocarcinoma of lung（bronchioloalveolar carcinoma）
癌细胞沿肺泡壁生长扩展，有乳头形成。肺泡间隔完整

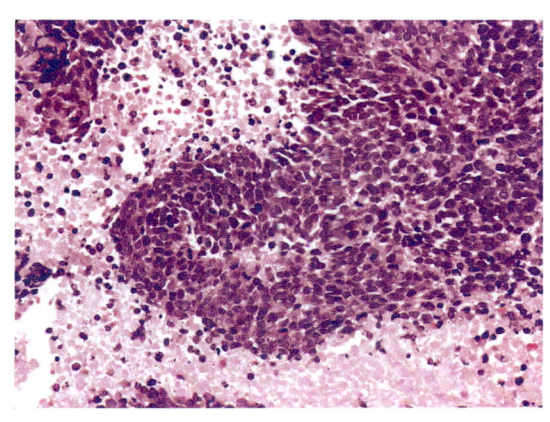

图 214 肺小细胞癌
Small cell carcinoma of lung
癌细胞体积小，呈梭形，胞浆少，裸核状，似燕麦，细胞排列呈片状，周围有坏死

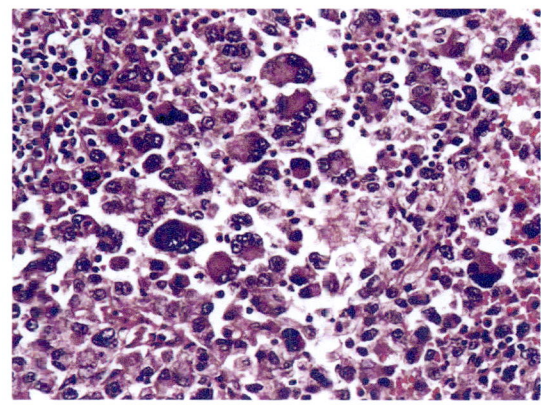

图 215 肺大细胞癌
Large cell carcinoma of lung
癌细胞体积大，核大深染，异型性明显。胞浆丰富，均质粉染。可见大量瘤巨细胞

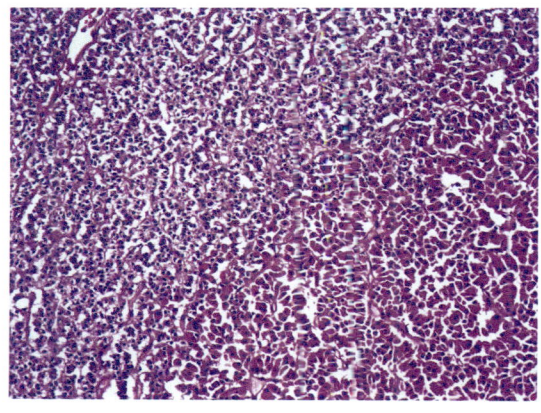

图 216 肺类癌
Carcinoid of lung
癌细胞呈条索或片块状排列，细胞大小形态较为一致，胞核位于中央。部分癌细胞胞浆透明，部分呈嗜酸性

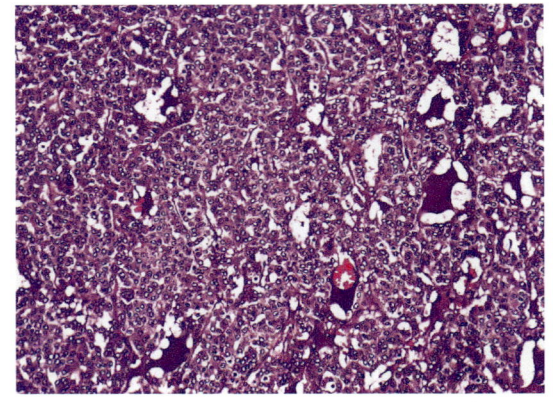

图217 肺类癌
Carcinoid of lung
癌细胞排列紧密，呈条索或腺泡样。细胞大小较一致，间质中见较多薄壁血管

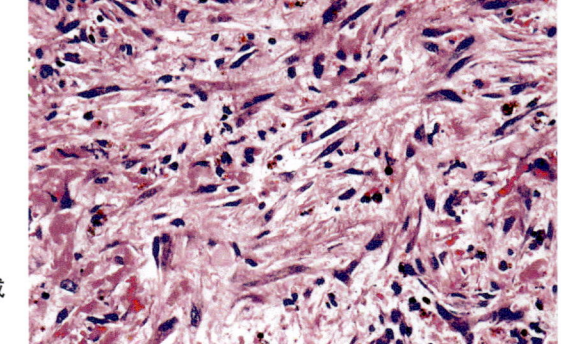

图218 胸膜间皮瘤
Pleural mesothelioma
瘤细胞排列成束状，瘤细胞形态似成纤维细胞

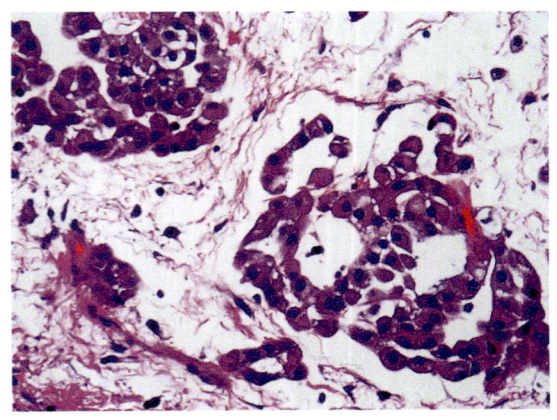

图219 胸膜间皮瘤
Pleural mesothelioma
与图218为同一肿瘤。瘤细胞形成腺腔样结构，显示该肿瘤的双向分化

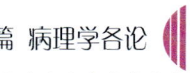

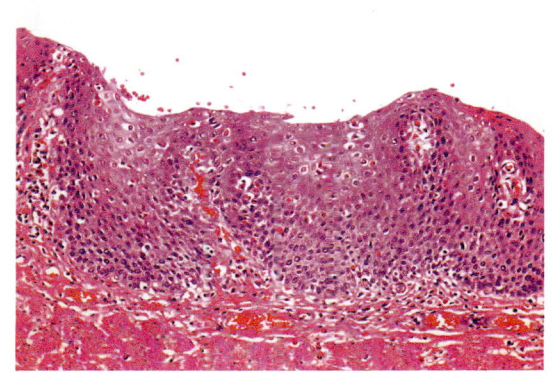

图 220　反流性食管炎
Regurgitant esophagitis
食管黏膜充血、水肿，淋巴细胞、浆细胞等炎细胞浸润

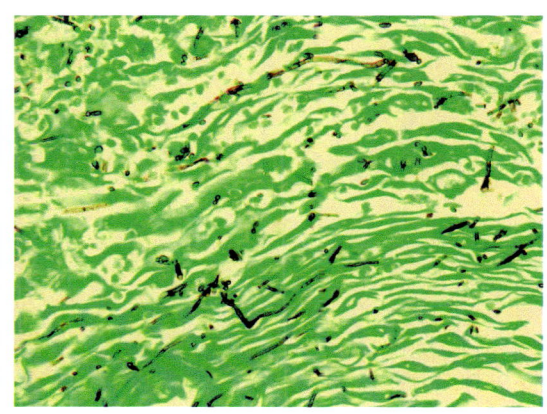

图 221　白色念珠菌食管炎
Candida albicans esophagitis
白色念珠菌的芽生孢子和假菌丝侵入食管黏膜下层和肌层，为银浸染色

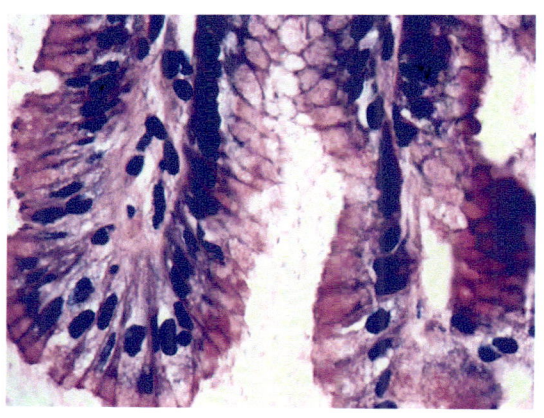

图 222　幽门螺杆菌性胃炎
H. pylori gastritis
胃黏膜充血、水肿，表浅上皮坏死脱落，固有层内淋巴细胞、浆细胞等炎细胞浸润

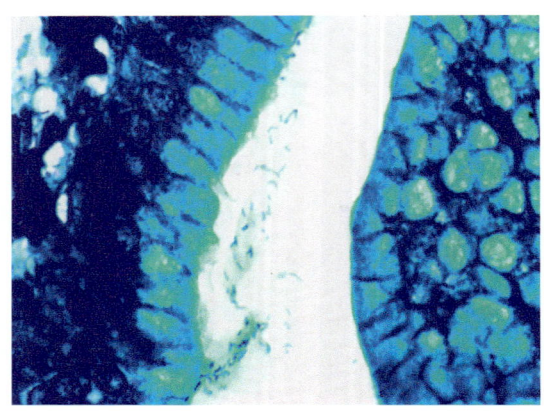

图223 幽门螺杆菌性胃炎
（Giemsa 染色）
H. pylori gastritis
胃黏膜上皮表面可见弯曲、螺旋形的幽门螺杆菌

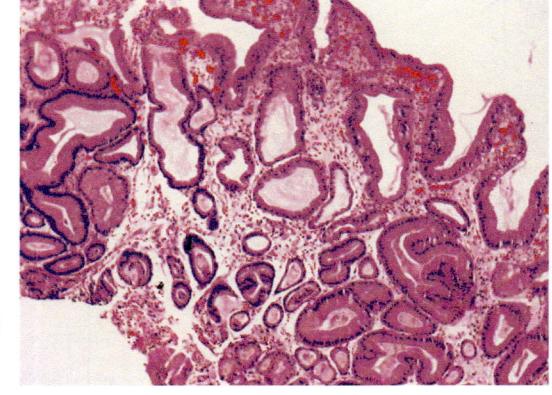

图224 慢性萎缩性胃炎
Chronic atrophic gastritis
胃黏膜萎缩变薄，腺体减少，固有层内淋巴细胞、浆细胞浸润

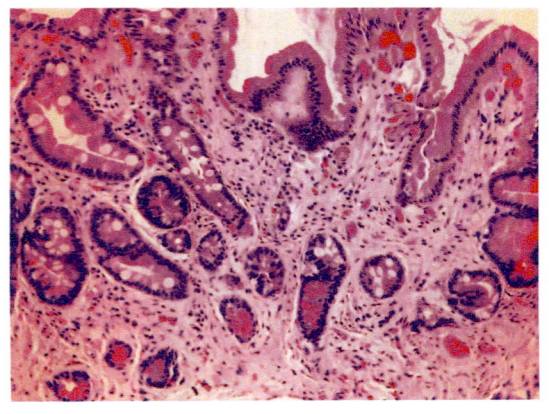

图225 胃肠上皮化生
Intestinal metaplasia of stomach
胃黏膜腺体萎缩，腺上皮中出现分泌黏液的杯状细胞

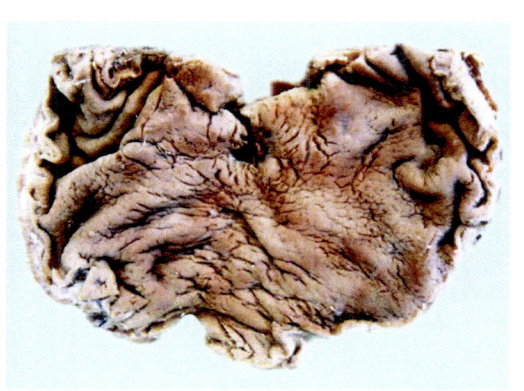

图 226 胃溃疡
Gastric ulcer
胃小弯近幽门部出现类圆形组织缺损，边缘整齐，底部平坦，黏膜皱襞向周围放射状排列

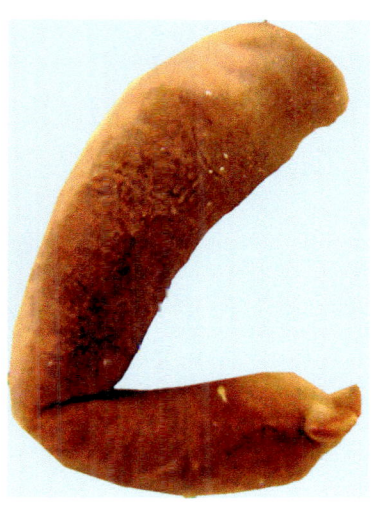

图 227 急性化脓性阑尾炎
Acute suppurative appendicitis
阑尾显著肿胀，浆膜充血，表面有脓性纤维素渗出

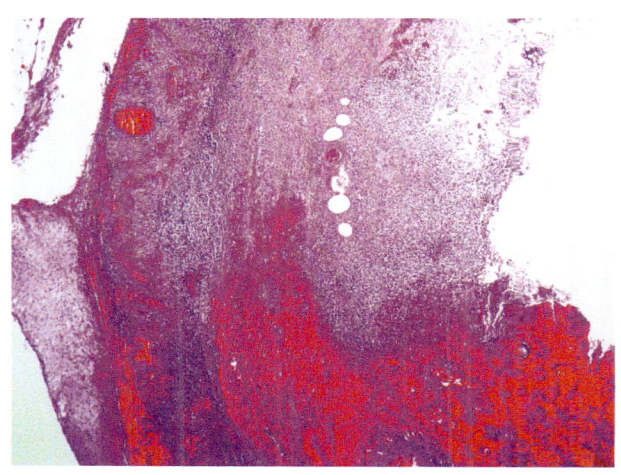

图 228 急性化脓性阑尾炎
Acute suppurative appendicitis
阑尾黏膜上皮坏死、脱落，管壁各层弥漫性中性粒细胞浸润，出血严重

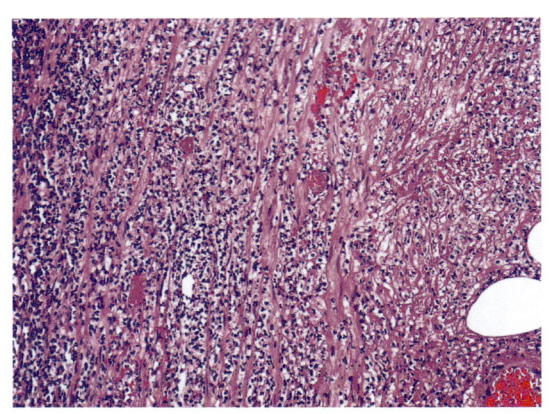

图229 急性化脓性阑尾炎
Acute suppurative appendicitis
阑尾炎性病变直达肌层及浆膜层，各层均有大量中性粒细胞弥漫浸润，伴炎性水肿

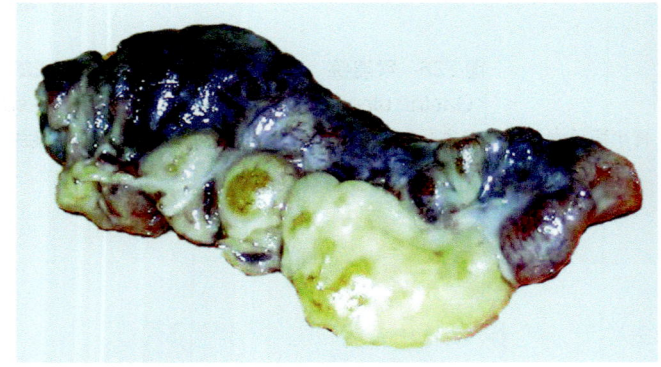

图230 急性坏疽性阑尾炎
Acute gangrenous appendicitis
阑尾肿胀，暗红色与黑色相间，部分有脓液覆盖

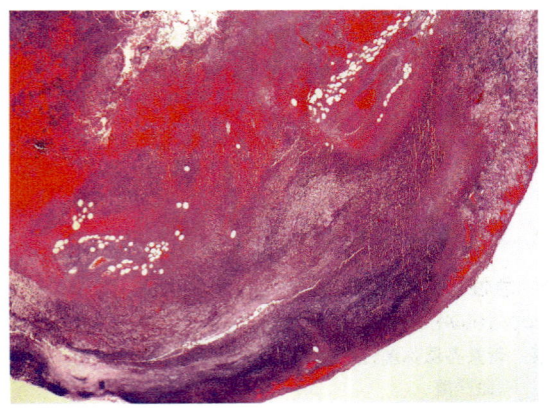

图231 急性坏疽性阑尾炎
Acute gangrenous appendicitis
阑尾壁坏死、出血明显，腔内阻塞，有脓性积液

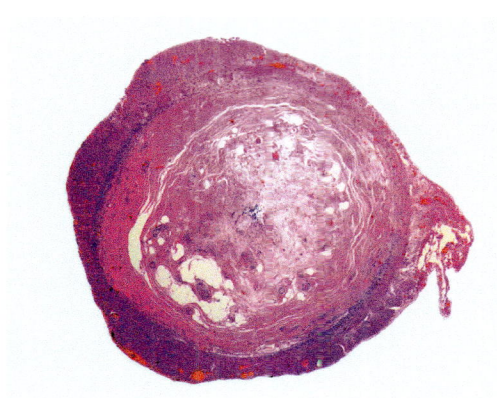

图 232 慢性阑尾炎
Chronic appendicitis
阑尾壁大量纤维成分增生，淋巴细胞、浆细胞等炎细胞浸润，管腔闭塞

图 233 Crohn 病
Crohn's disease
肠壁全层淋巴细胞、浆细胞、巨噬细胞浸润，大量淋巴组织增生，有结核样肉芽肿，黏膜下层有小血管扩张

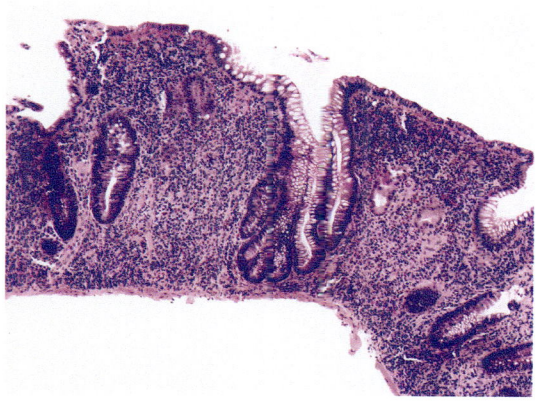

图 234 慢性溃疡性结肠炎
Chronic ulcerative colitis
肠壁局部小溃疡形成，黏膜及黏膜下层中粒细胞、淋巴细胞、嗜酸粒细胞等炎细胞浸润

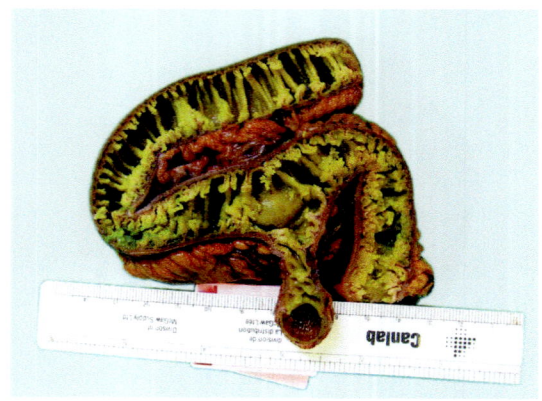

图 235　Meckel 憩室
Meckel's diverticulum
憩室呈指状膨出，位于肠系膜附着部的对侧，内壁有与回肠同样的黏膜

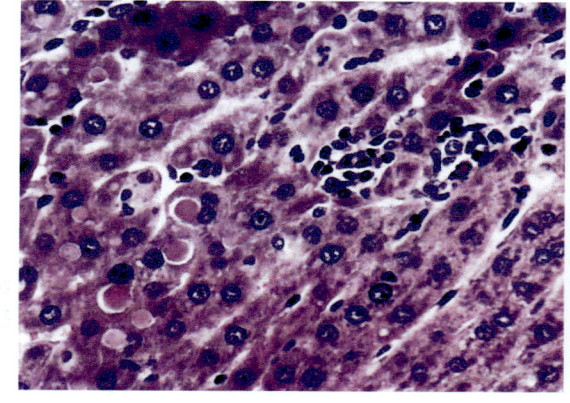

图 236　急性病毒性肝炎
Acute viral hepatitis
肝细胞广泛变性，体积增大，胞浆疏松化，嗜酸性变，点状坏死，肝窦受压变窄

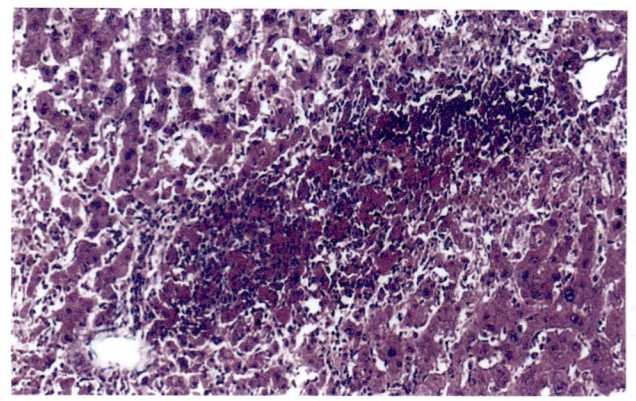

图 237　慢性肝炎，桥接坏死
Chronic hepatitis, bridging necrosis
肝小叶两个中央静脉之间出现互相连接的肝细胞坏死带，并伴有炎细胞浸润

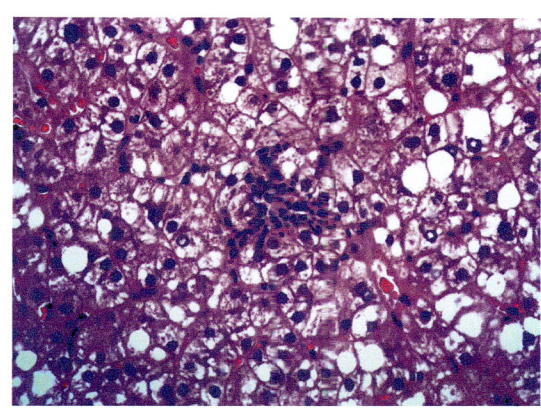

图 238　酒精性肝炎
Alcoholic hepatitis
肝细胞脂肪变性，灶状坏死伴中性粒细胞浸润

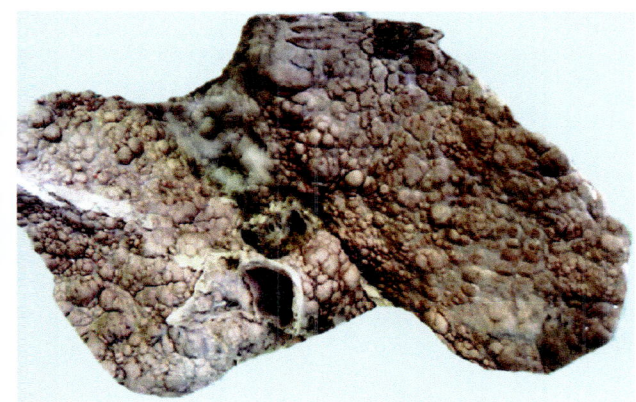

图 239　门脉性肝硬化
Portal cirrhosis
肝脏体积缩小，质地变硬，表面可见大小较一致的细小结节

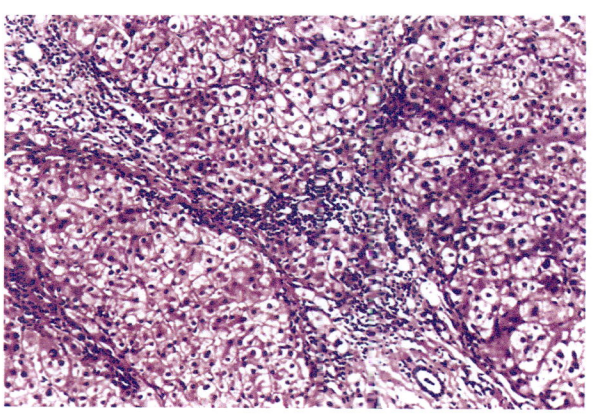

图 240　门脉性肝硬化
Portal cirrhosis
广泛增生的纤维组织将肝小叶重新分割包绕形成假小叶；假小叶为肝细胞变性、排列紊乱；纤维间隔内有淋巴细胞、单核细胞浸润，小胆管增生

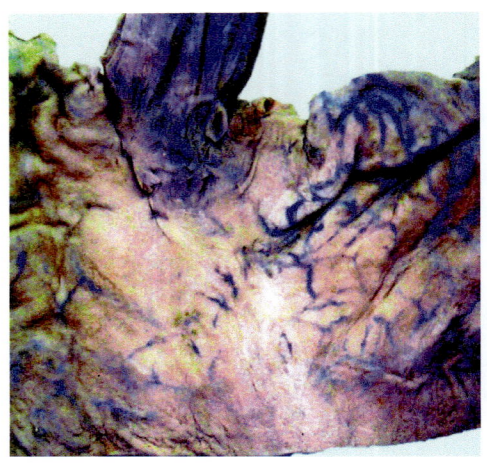

图241 食管下段静脉曲张
Esophageal varices
食管下段和胃连接处静脉曲张,突出于黏膜表面

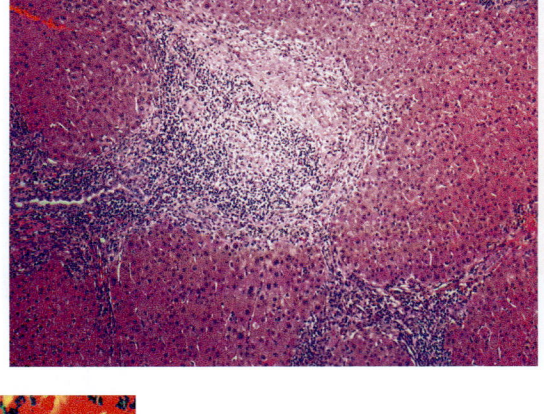

图242 原发性胆汁性肝硬化
Primary biliary cirrhosis
肝小叶间胆管上皮细胞坏死,淋巴细胞浸润,结缔组织增生并伸入肝小叶内,假小叶呈不完全分割型

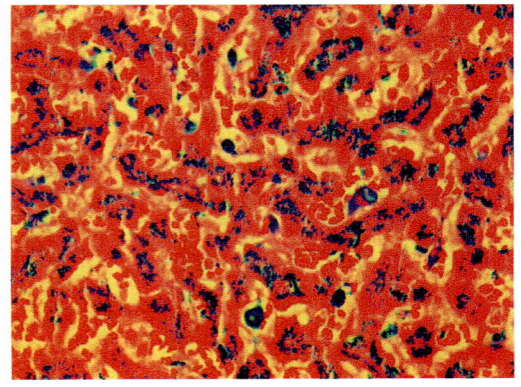

图243 肝血色病
Liver hemochromatosis
肝内重度含铁血黄素沉积,为普鲁士蓝改良染色

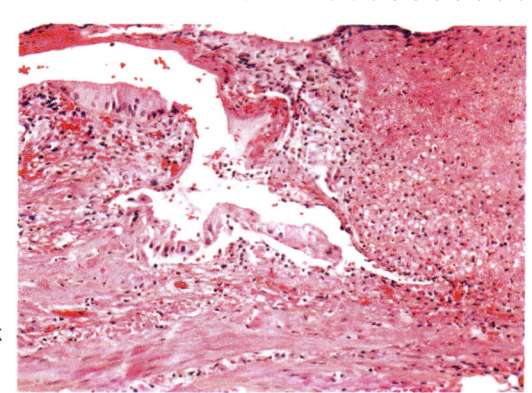

图 244　急性胆囊炎
Acute cholecystitis
胆囊黏膜充血、水肿，上皮细胞坏死脱落，囊壁有中性粒细胞浸润

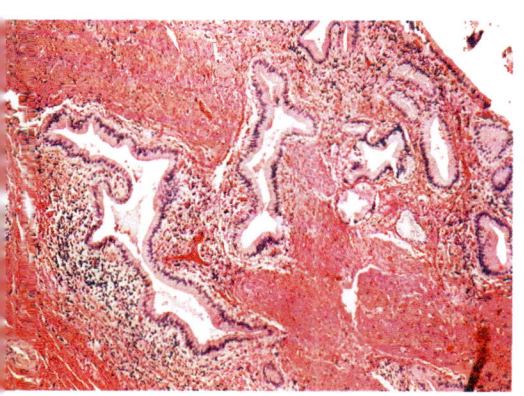

图 245　慢性胆囊炎
Chronic cholecystitis
胆囊黏膜萎缩，囊壁各层均有淋巴细胞、单核细胞浸润，纤维组织增生

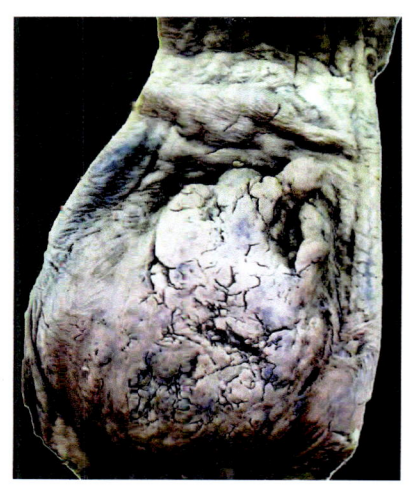

图 246　食管癌
Carcinoma of esophagus
癌呈灰白色扁平肿块，突向食管腔

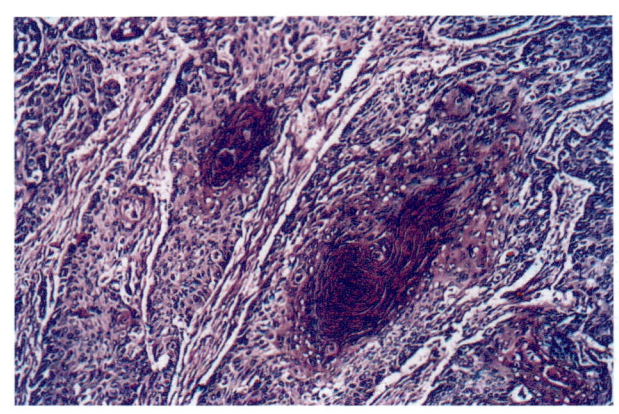

图247 食管鳞癌
Squamous cell carcinoma of esophagus
癌组织为高分化鳞癌，可见癌巢结构，中间有角化珠，实质和间质区分清楚

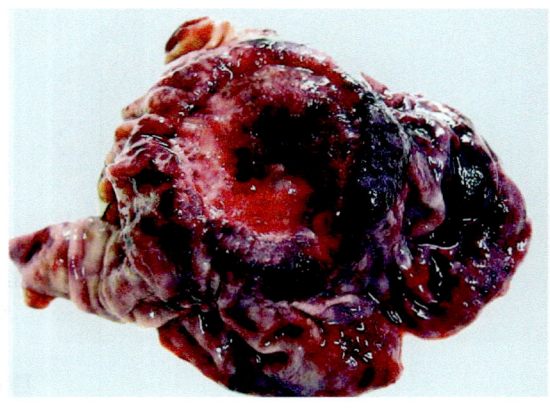

图248 溃疡型胃癌
Ulcerative type of gastric carcinoma
癌组织坏死脱落形成溃疡，较大、边缘隆起、界限不清，底部凹凸不平

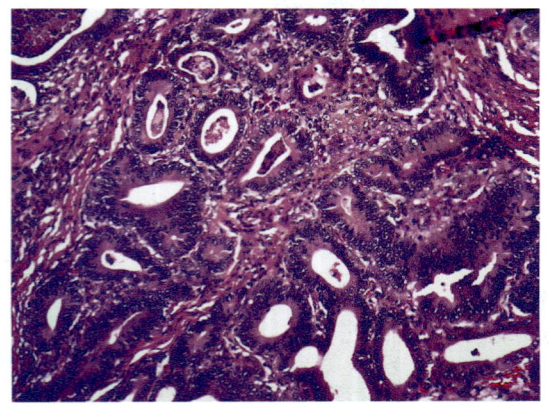

图249 胃腺癌
Adenocarcinoma of stomach
癌细胞形成明显的管腔结构，管腔形状、大小不一，细胞异型性明显

第2篇 病理学各论

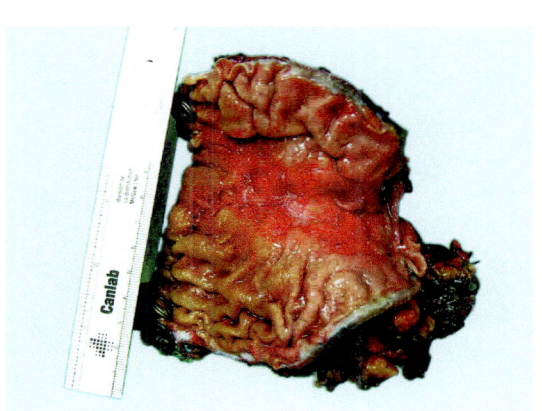

图 250 弥漫性浸润型胃癌
Diffuse invasive type of gastric carcinoma
癌组织向胃壁内弥漫浸润，与周围正常组织界限不清，表面黏膜皱襞大部分消失，可见浅表溃疡

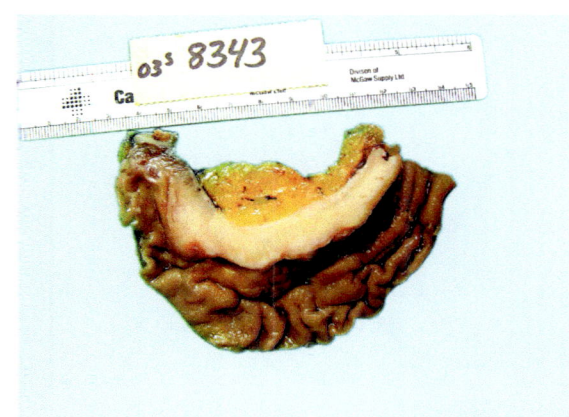

图 251 弥漫性浸润型胃癌
Diffuse invasive type of gastric carcinoma
癌组织沿胃壁弥漫浸润，与周围正常组织界限不清

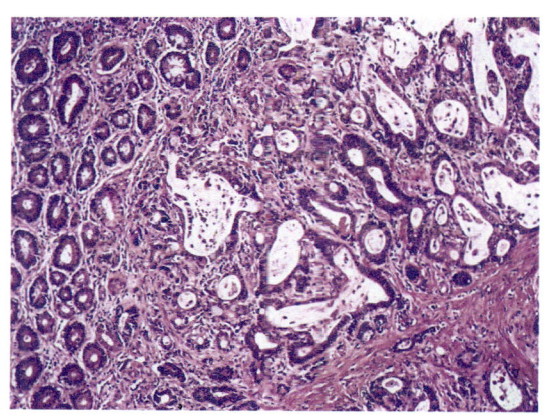

图 252 胃腺癌
Adenocarcinoma of stomach
癌组织有清楚的腺样结构，排列紊乱，浸润到肌层，细胞分化不一

85

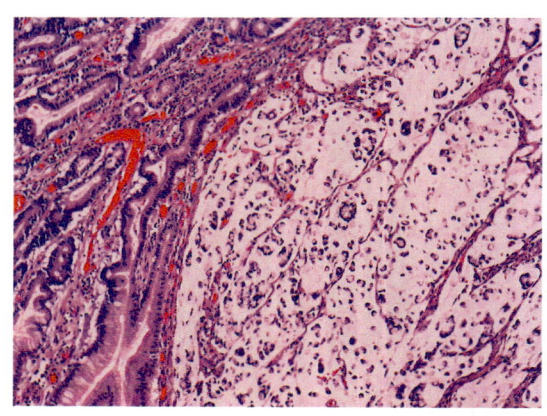

图253　胃黏液癌（低倍镜）
Mucinous carcinoma of stomach
癌组织内有大量黏液积聚，形成黏液湖，癌细胞成片或单个位于其中，胞浆淡染

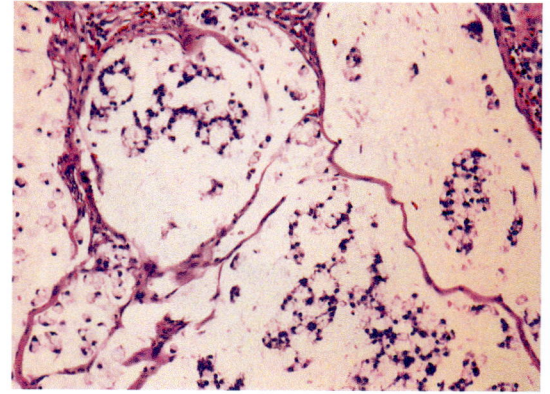

图254　胃黏液癌（高倍镜）
Mucinous carcinoma of stomach
成团或单个的癌细胞漂浮于黏液湖中，有的单个癌细胞呈印戒状

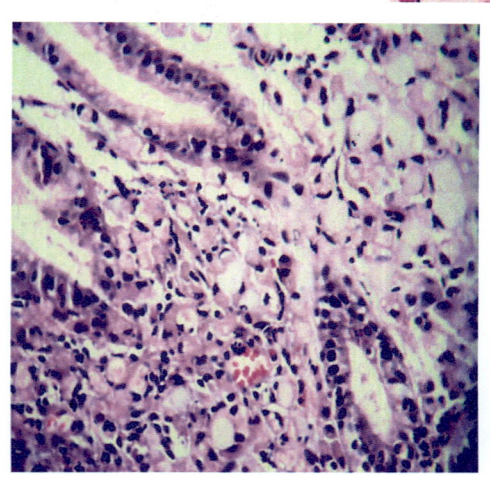

图255　胃印戒细胞癌
Signet-ring cell carcinoma of stomach
癌细胞呈分散性浸润，细胞圆形，由于分泌大量黏液而将核挤压到细胞一侧，形如戒指

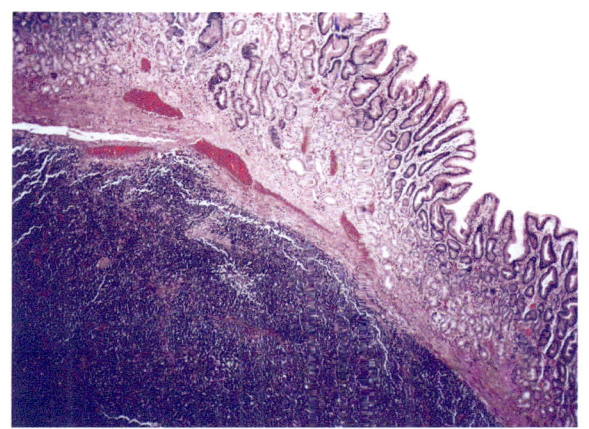

图 256 胃小细胞癌（低倍镜）
Small cell carcinoma of stomach
癌组织呈实性生长，间质血管丰富，可见坏死，细胞圆形或梭形，胞浆少

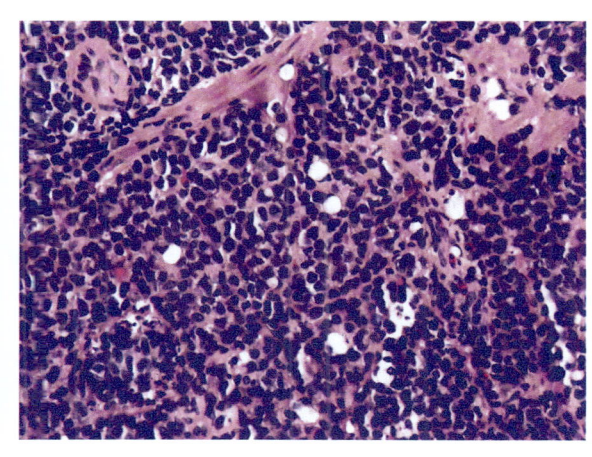

图 257 胃小细胞癌（高倍镜）
Small cell carcinoma of stomach
癌细胞体积较小，圆形或梭形，胞浆稀少，核形态规则，浓染，核仁不明显

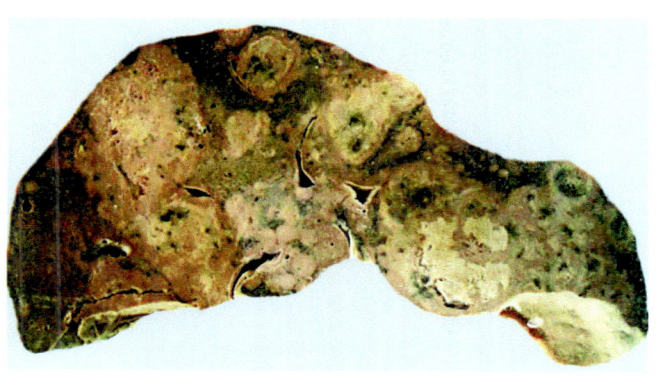

图 258 胃癌肝转移
Metastatic gastric carcinoma in liver
肝脏可见多个灰白色肿块，有的互相融合，表面可见出血、坏死

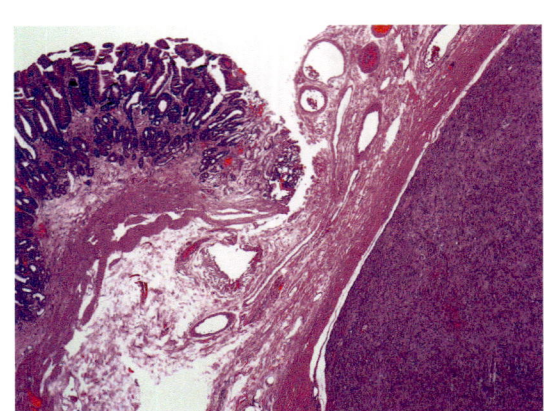

图 259 胃平滑肌瘤（低倍镜）
Leiomyoma of stomach
瘤组织位于黏膜下，与周围组织境界清楚，瘤细胞较密集

图 260 胃平滑肌瘤（高倍镜）
Leiomyoma of stomach
肿瘤由分化成熟的平滑肌细胞组成，胞浆丰富，嗜酸性，呈束状平行排列，间质可见玻璃样变性

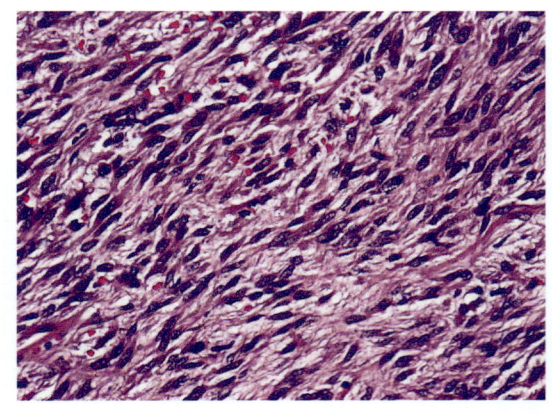

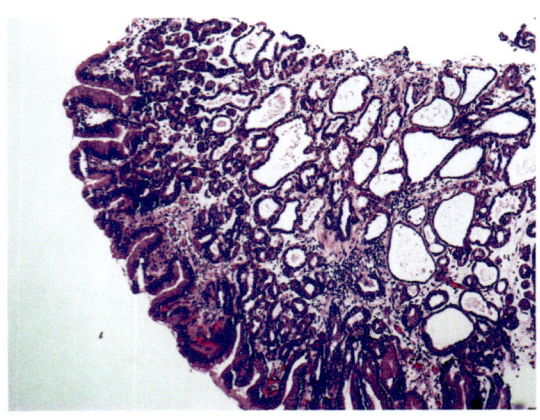

图 261 胃底腺息肉
Fundic gland polyp
息肉内腺体呈囊状扩张，内衬覆胃底腺上皮，混有正常的腺体，间质有慢性炎细胞浸润

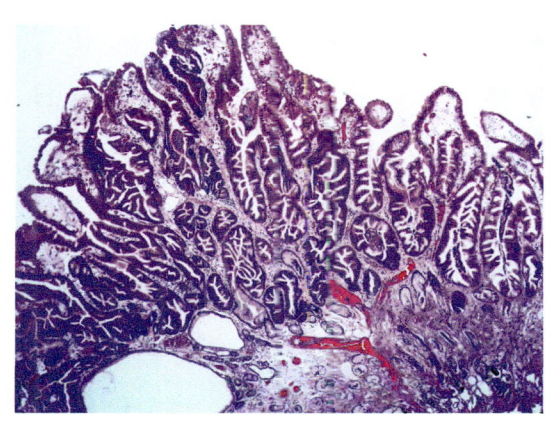

图262 胃增生性息肉
Hyperplastic polyp of stomach
息肉内腺体呈囊状和不规则分支，内衬覆单层增生的小凹型上皮，间质水肿，浆细胞、淋巴细胞等浸润

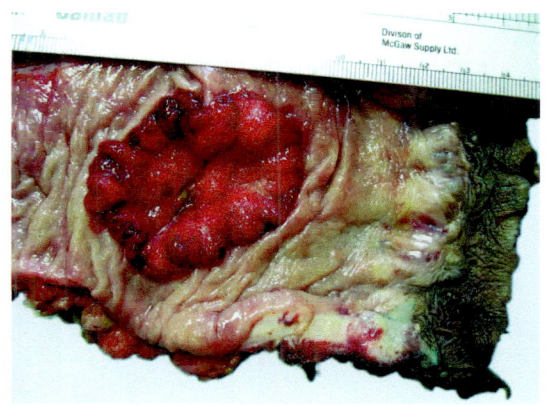

图263 溃疡型直肠癌
Ulcerative type of rectal carcinoma
肿瘤表面形成较深溃疡，呈火山口状，边缘隆起、外翻，底部凹凸不平

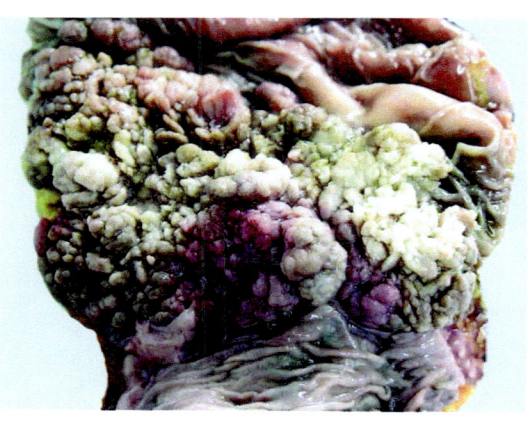

图264 隆起型肠癌
Massive type of intestinal carcinoma
肿瘤呈息肉状向肠腔突出，表面不坏脱落，有浅表溃疡

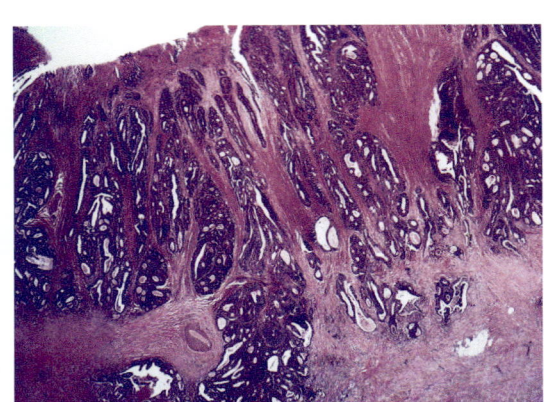

图 265　结肠腺癌（低倍镜）
Adenocarcinoma of colon
癌组织形成腺管样结构，大小形态不一

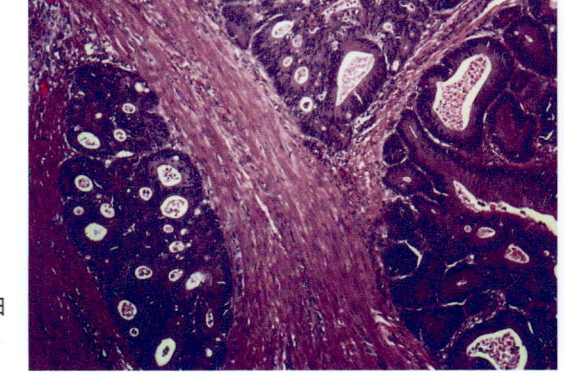

图 266　结肠腺癌（高倍镜）
Adenocarcinoma of colon
癌细胞围成腺管状，形状不规则，细胞异型性明显

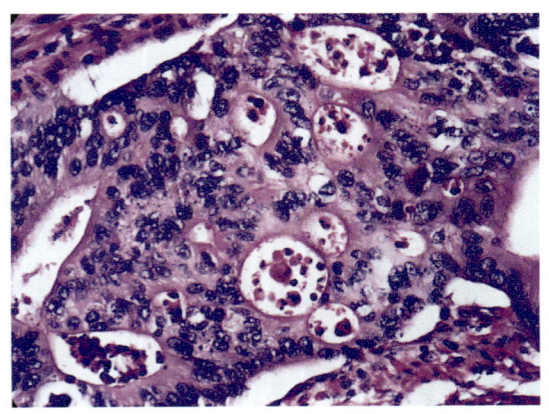

图 267　结肠腺癌凋亡
Apoptosis of colon adenocarcinoma cells
癌细胞核大，染色不均，可见凋亡现象

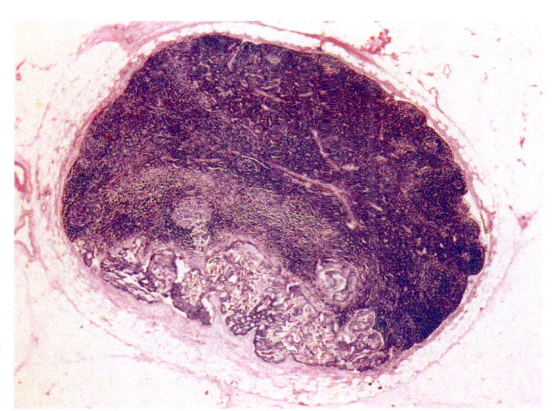

图268 结肠腺癌淋巴结转移
Metastatic colon adenocarcinoma in lymph node
淋巴结边缘窦可见癌组织，排列成形态不规则的腺管样结构

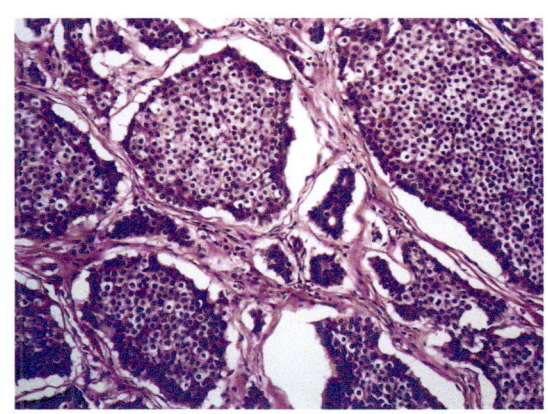

图269 小肠类癌
Carcinoid tumor of small bowel
癌细胞排列紧密呈团块状、实心岛状，细胞大小一致，呈小圆形或卵圆形，胞浆少呈颗粒状，弱嗜酸性

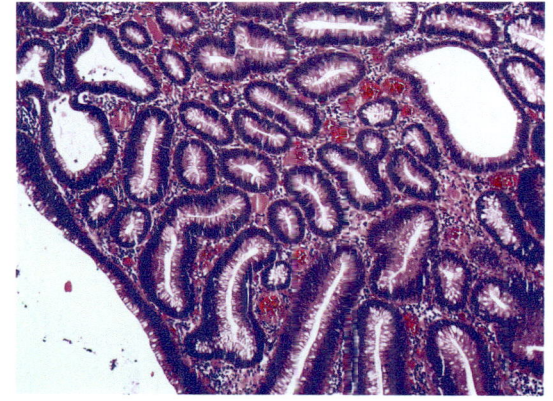

图270 结肠管状腺瘤
Tubular adenoma of colon
肿瘤由管状结构构成，形态不一，表面被覆不典型增生的上皮

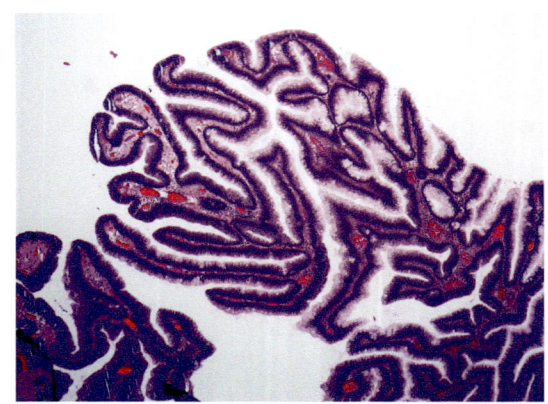

图271 结肠绒毛状腺瘤
Villus adenoma of colon
肿瘤为固有膜形成的分叶状突起，表面被覆轻度不典型增生的上皮

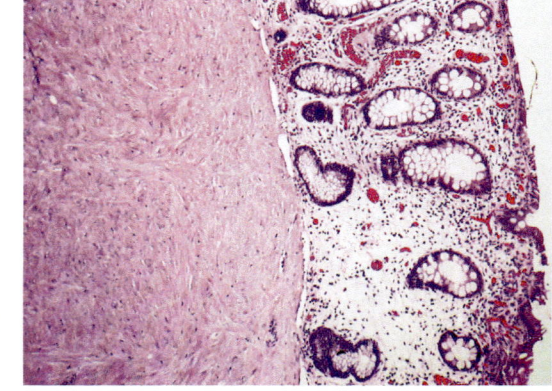

图272 直肠平滑肌瘤
Leiomyoma of rectum
瘤组织界限清楚，由编织样排列的分化较好的平滑肌细胞组成

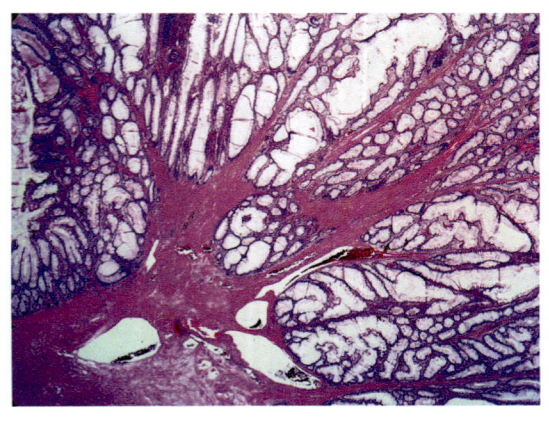

图273 结肠 Peutz-Jephers 息肉
Peutz-Jephers polyp of colon
息肉由分化良好的腺上皮构成，腺体呈分支状，排列紊乱，腺腔可轻度扩张，腺管排列紧密，间质少，炎症反应不明显；黏膜肌增生呈树枝状穿插于腺管之间

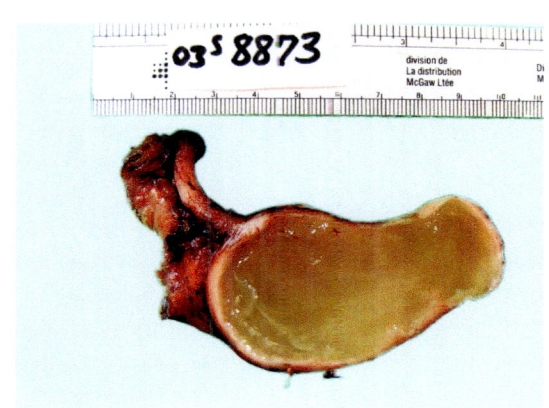

图274 阑尾黏液囊腺瘤
Mucinous cystadenoma of appendix
阑尾呈囊性扩张，腔内可见大量胶冻样黏液

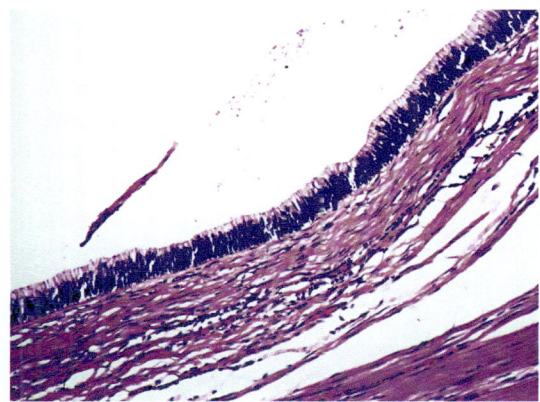

图275 阑尾黏液囊腺瘤
Mucinous cystadenoma of appendix
囊腺瘤腺腔高度扩张，充满黏液，内衬柱状上皮

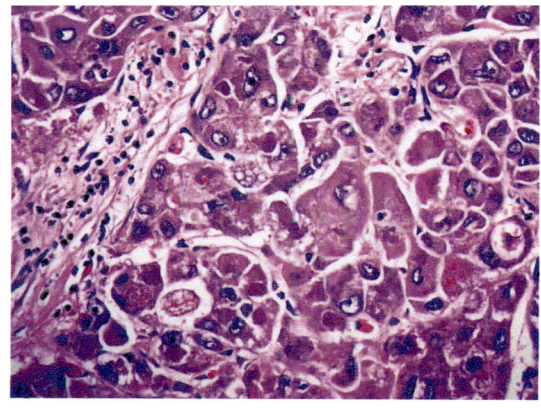

图276 肝细胞癌
Hepatocellular carcinoma
癌细胞胞浆丰富，颗粒状，嗜伊红染，胞核较大，核膜厚，染色质集中于核膜周围，核仁大而明显，有淤胆现象

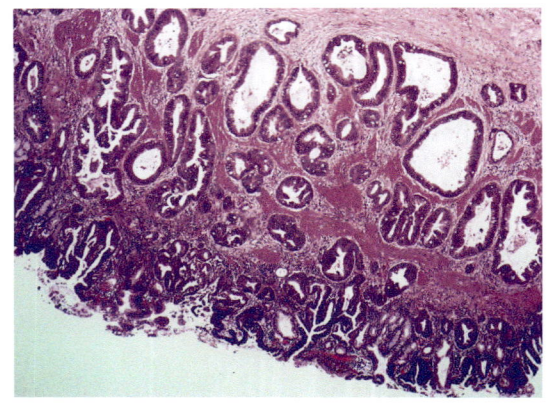

图 277 胆囊腺癌
Adenocarcinoma of gallbladder
癌组织形成腺样结构，轮廓不整齐，间质纤维结缔组织丰富，癌细胞呈柱状，分化较好

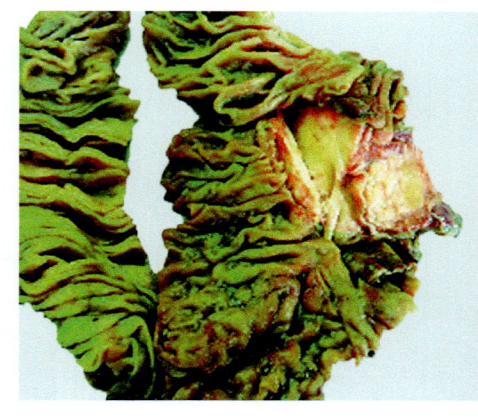

图 278 胰头癌
Carcinoma of head of pancreas
肿瘤体积较小，切面灰白色和黄白色相间，可见少量出血

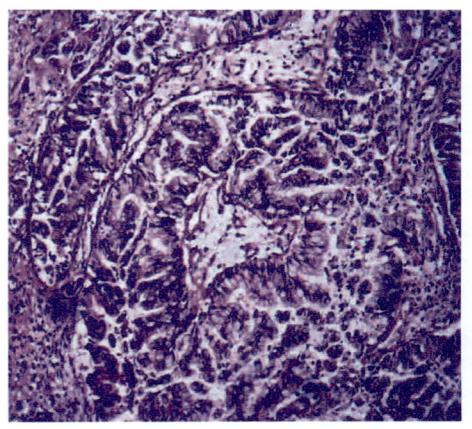

图 279 胰腺导管腺癌
Ductal adenocarcinoma of pancreas
肿瘤组织由分化较差的腺管构成，腺管不规则，有的为小的实性团，间质丰富，细胞异型性明显

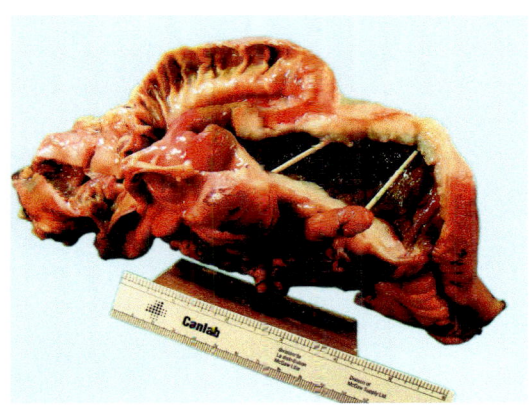

图 280 弥漫性大 B 细胞淋巴瘤
（远端回肠）
Diffuse large-B cell lymphoma
(distal ileum)
肿瘤组织弥漫浸润，导致肠壁增厚，结构不清。瘤组织质地细腻、湿润

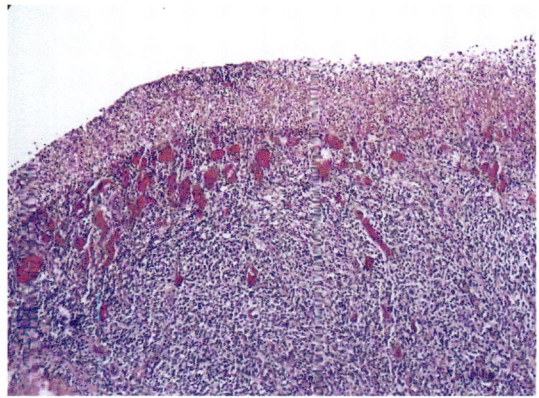

图 281 弥漫性大 B 细胞淋巴瘤
（远端回肠）
Diffuse large-B cell lymphoma
(distal ileum)
肠黏膜表层坏死，黏膜下见肿瘤组织弥漫增生

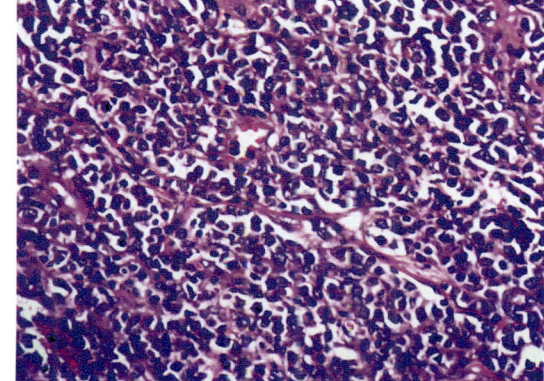

图 282 弥漫性大 B 细胞淋巴瘤
Diffuse large-B cell lymphoma
弥漫浸润的瘤细胞体积大，胞浆丰富。核圆或椭圆形，大部分细胞核仁明显

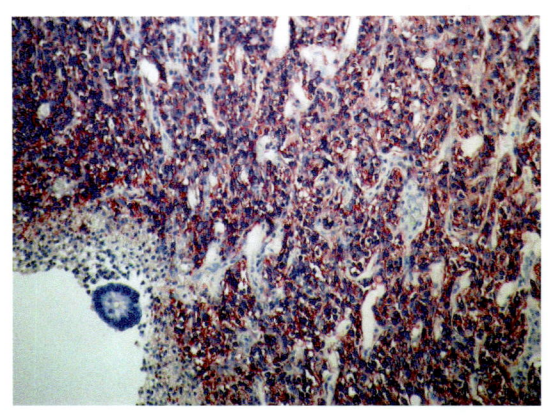

图283 弥漫性大B细胞淋巴瘤
Diffuse large-B cell lymphoma
免疫组化染色显示，几乎全部瘤细胞CD20膜阳性。证明其B细胞来源

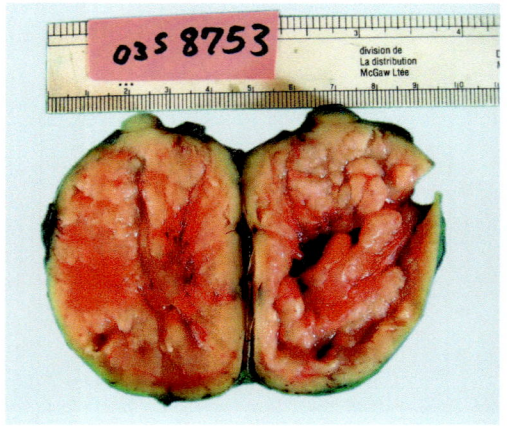

图284 弥漫性大B细胞淋巴瘤（腋下淋巴结）
Diffuse large-B cell lymphoma (axillary lymph node)
淋巴结肿大，切面结构不清，质地细腻似鱼肉状

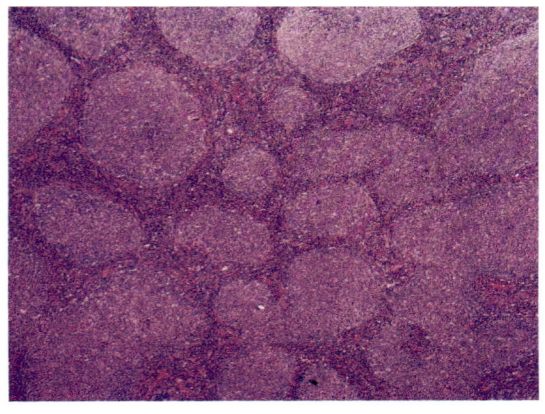

图285 滤泡性淋巴瘤（颈部淋巴结）
Follicular lymphoma (cervical lymph node)
淋巴结正常结构消失，代之以构成滤泡样结构的肿瘤组织。肿瘤性滤泡排列紧密，缺乏套区

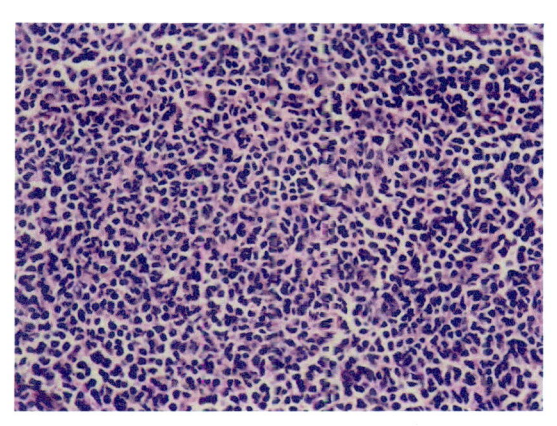

图286 滤泡性淋巴瘤(1级)
Follicular lymphoma (grade 1)
肿瘤细胞呈滤泡中心细胞样，核不规则，有棱角，无明显核仁。无中心母细胞

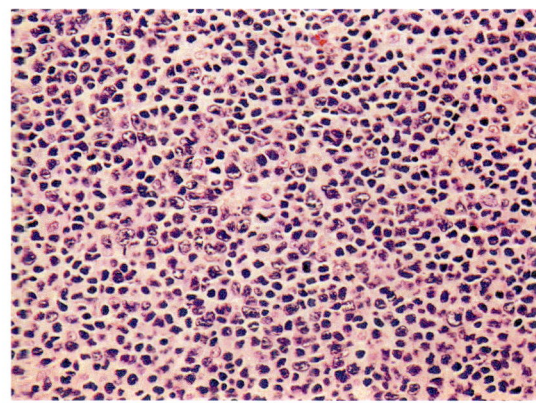

图287 滤泡性淋巴瘤(2级)
Follicular lymphoma (grade 2)
肿瘤组织由大、中、小肿瘤细胞混合组成。较小的肿瘤细胞似中心细胞。中等及大者似中心母细胞，核圆形泡状，有1~3个位于核膜下的核仁

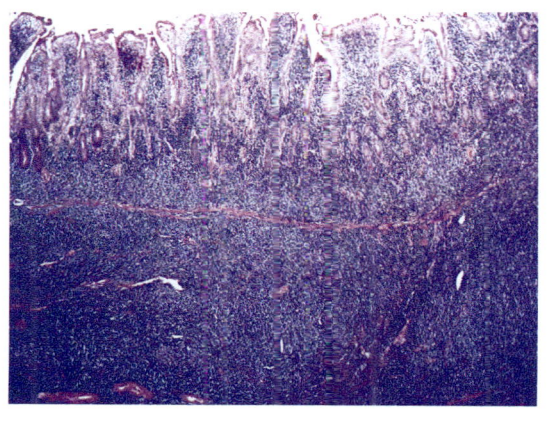

图288 黏膜相关淋巴组织
(MALT)淋巴瘤
Mucosa-associated lymphoid tissue lymphoma
肿瘤细胞弥漫浸润于(小肠)黏膜及黏膜下各层

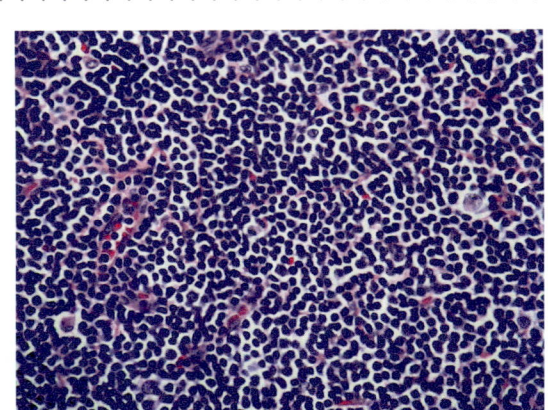

图289 黏膜相关淋巴组织
（MALT）淋巴瘤
Mucosa-associated lymphoid
tissue lymphoma
肿瘤细胞类似小淋巴细胞，伴散在转化的母细胞

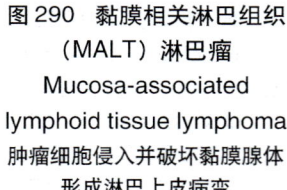

图290 黏膜相关淋巴组织
（MALT）淋巴瘤
Mucosa-associated
lymphoid tissue lymphoma
肿瘤细胞侵入并破坏黏膜腺体形成淋巴上皮病变

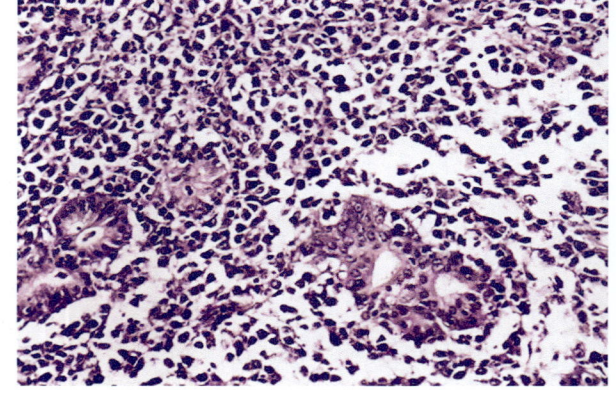

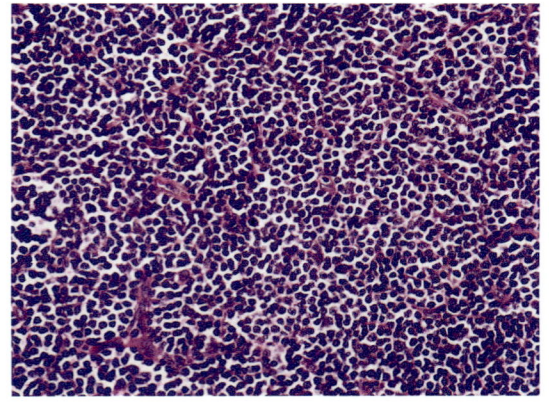

图291 慢性淋巴细胞性白血病/
小细胞性淋巴瘤病
Chronic lymphocytic leukaemia/
small lymphocytic lymphoma
肿瘤细胞增生呈片状，细胞体积小，胞浆少，核染色质凝集成块状，并有单个小核仁

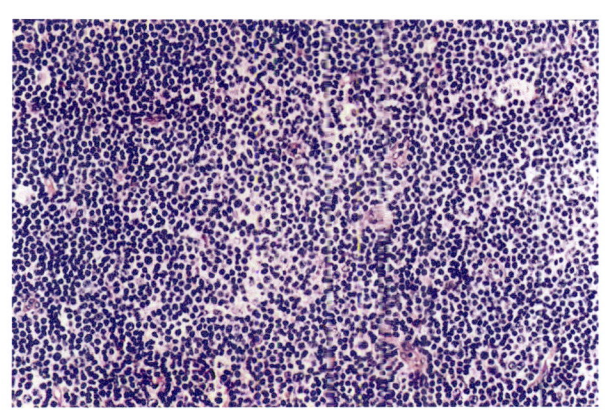

图292 慢性淋巴细胞性白血病/小细胞性淋巴瘤病
Chronic lymphocytic leukaemia/small lymphocytic lymphoma
片状肿瘤细胞中见浅染的增殖中心,其内有副免疫母细胞,此细胞体积较大,核圆或椭圆形,内见中位小核仁

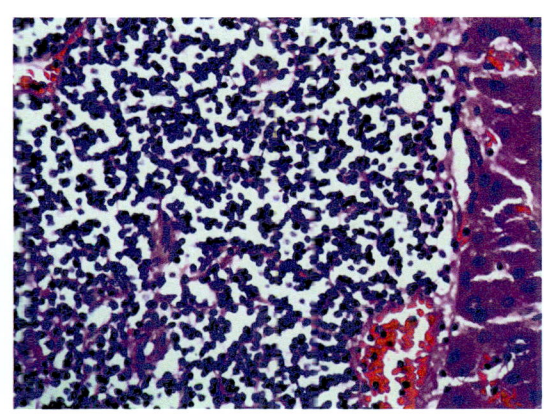

图293 慢性淋巴细胞性白血病/小细胞性淋巴瘤病
Chronic lymphocytic leukaemia/small lymphocytic lymphoma
小淋巴细胞样肿瘤细胞在肝脏组织内结节性浸润

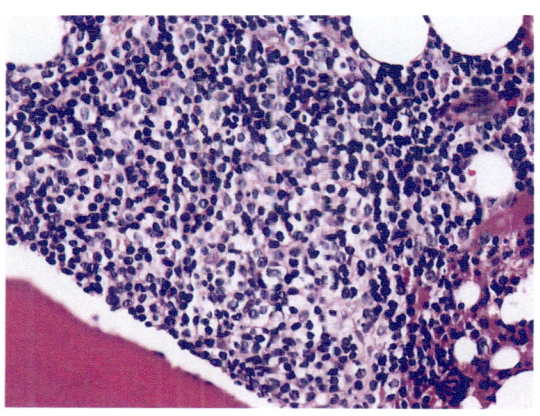

图294 套细胞淋巴瘤(骨)
Mantle cell lymphoma (bone)
肿瘤细胞弥漫片状浸润于骨组织,瘤细胞似淋巴母细胞,染色质细腻,内有小核仁

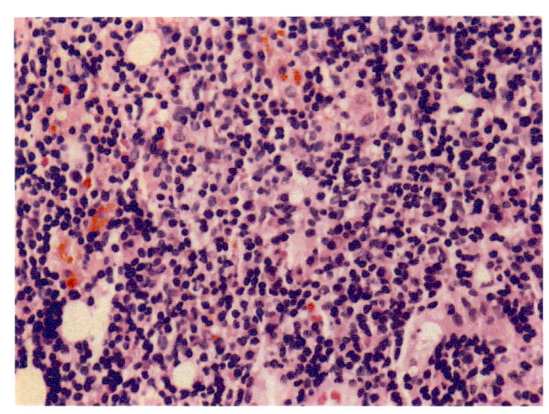

图295 淋巴浆细胞性淋巴瘤
Lymphoplasmacytic lymphoma
肿瘤组织由小淋巴细胞、浆细胞样淋巴细胞及浆细胞混合构成

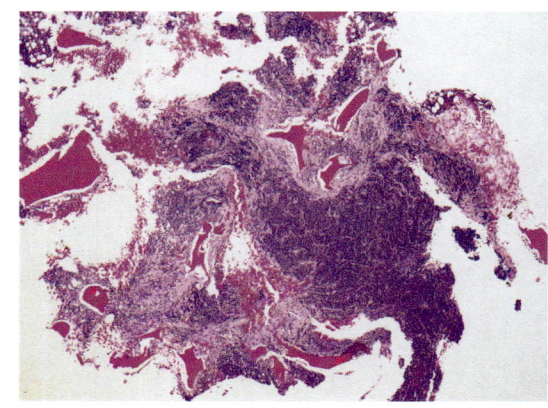

图296 多发性骨髓瘤
Multiple myeloma
肿瘤组织弥漫片状浸润骨髓组织

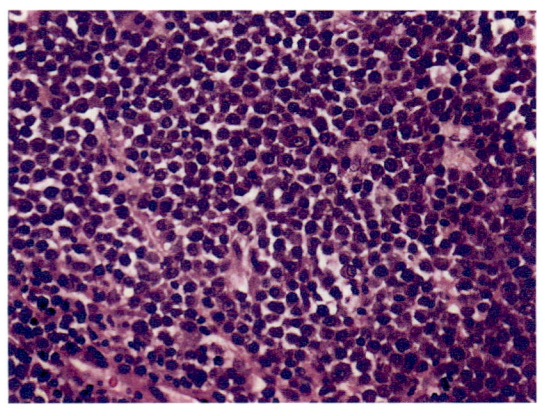

图297 多发性骨髓瘤
Multiple myeloma
图296高倍图。肿瘤细胞似浆细胞，细胞大小一致，胞浆嗜碱性，核偏位，染色质排列如车辐状

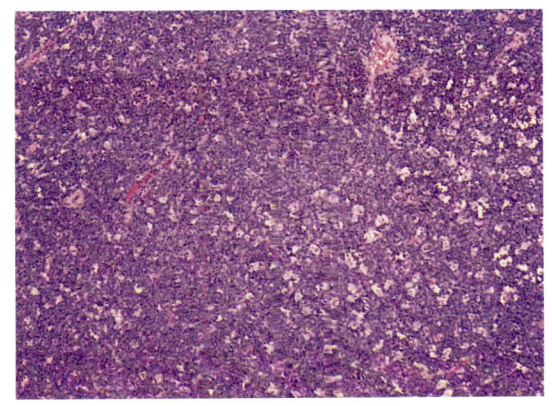

图 298　Burkitt 样淋巴瘤
Burkitt-like lymphoma
肿瘤组织由形态较一致的瘤细胞构成，内见散在巨噬细胞，构成星空现象

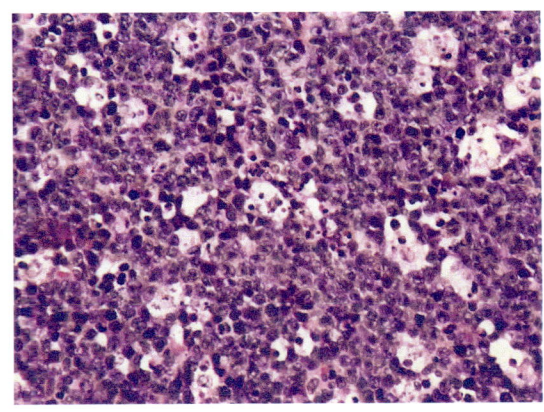

图 299　Burkitt 样淋巴瘤
Burkitt-like lymphoma
图 298 高倍图。肿瘤细胞中等大小，核形态不规则、多形，核仁明显，核分裂象较多，细胞凋亡多见。散在的巨噬细胞内有被吞噬细胞碎片

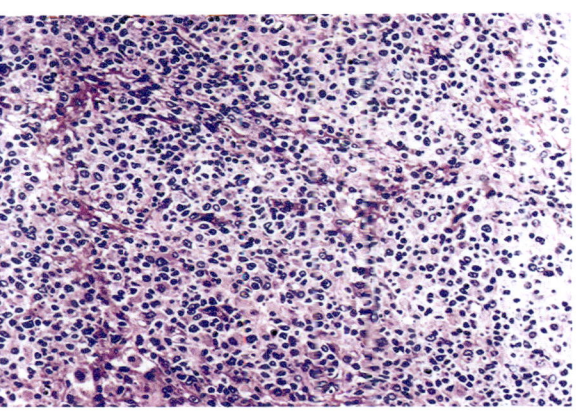

图 300　外周 T 细胞淋巴瘤（非特异性）
Peripheral T-cell lymphoma (unspecified)
肿瘤细胞由大小不等的多形性细胞组成。细胞浆多少不等、淡染。核呈多形性（北京大学医学部高子芬教授赠图）

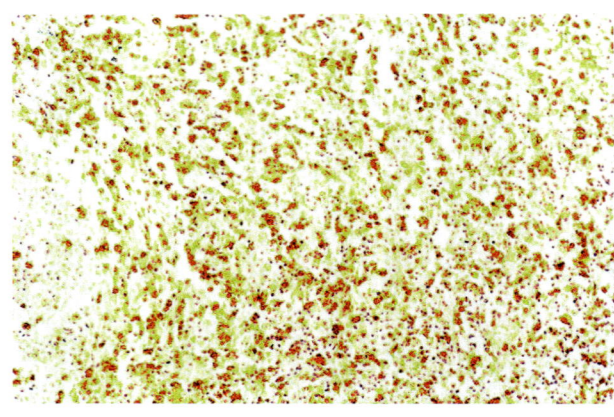

图 301　外周 T 细胞淋巴瘤（非特异性）
Peripheral T-cell lymphoma（unspecified）
免疫组化染色显示，几乎全部瘤细胞 CD3 阳性，证实其 T 细胞来源（北京大学医学部高子芬教授赠图）

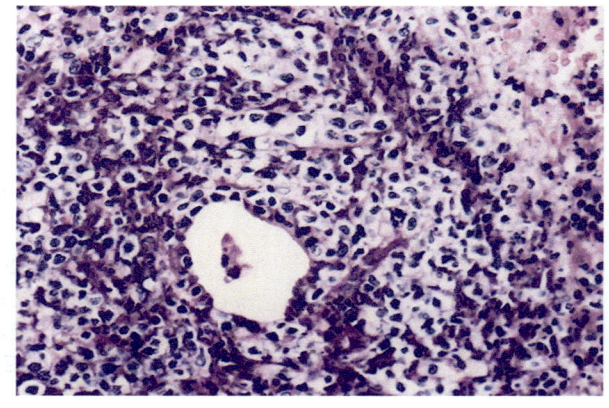

图 302　NK/T 细胞淋巴瘤
NK/T-cell lymphoma
肿瘤细胞中等大小，胞浆淡染，核多形，染色质细，核仁不明显。瘤细胞浸润破坏血管壁。图右侧可见坏死肿瘤组织（北京大学医学部高子芬教授赠图）

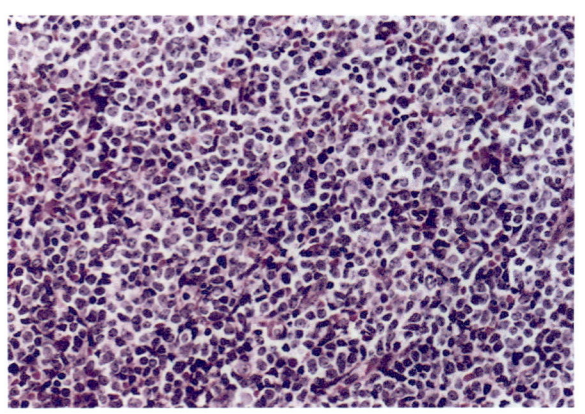

图 303　T 淋巴母细胞性淋巴瘤
T-lymphoblastic lymphoma
弥漫增生的肿瘤细胞中等大小，核圆或椭圆形，染色质呈细颗粒状，内见小核仁（北京大学医学部高子芬教授赠图）

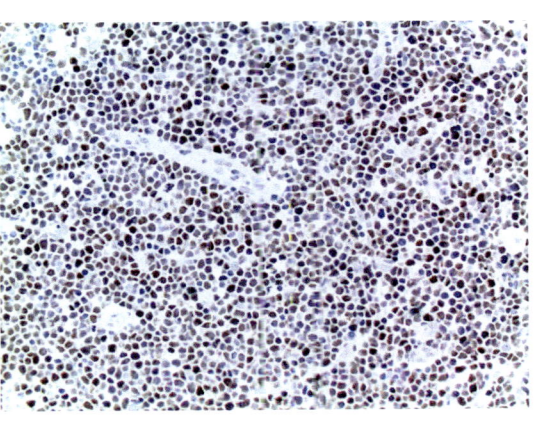

图 304 T 淋巴母细胞性淋巴瘤
T-lymphoblastic lymphoma
免疫组化染色显示，几乎所有肿瘤细胞表达 TdT，表明其来源于前淋巴细胞（北京大学医学部高子芬教授赠图）

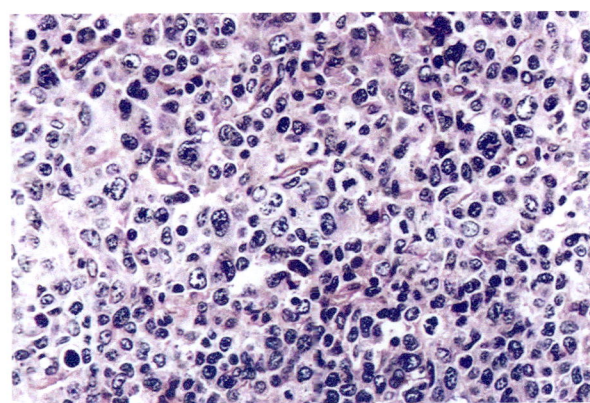

图 305 间变性大细胞淋巴瘤
Anaplastic large cell lymphoma
肿瘤细胞弥漫性增生，其中可见本型淋巴瘤的标志性细胞：体积大、胞浆丰富、偏位肾形核的细胞。核分裂较多（北京大学医学部高子芬教授赠图）

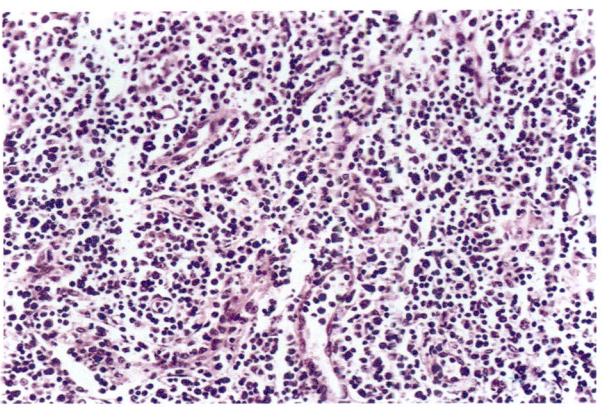

图 306 血管免疫母细胞性 T 细胞淋巴瘤
Angioimmunoblastic T-cell lymphoma
淋巴结结构消失，中等到较大的淋巴样细胞弥漫浸润。血管呈树枝状增生（北京大学医学部高子芬教授赠图）

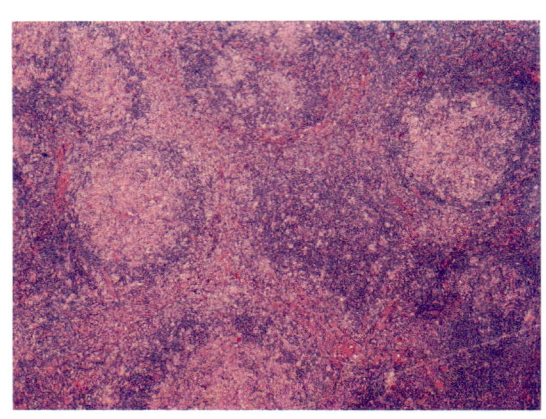

图307　结节性淋巴细胞为主型霍奇金淋巴瘤
Nodular lymphocyte predominant Hodgkin lymphoma
淋巴结正常结构消失，代之以紧密排列的结节样病灶

图308　结节性淋巴细胞为主型霍奇金淋巴瘤
Nodular lymphocyte predominant Hodgkin lymphoma
图307高倍图。显示结节内小淋巴细胞和组织细胞背景中较大的肿瘤细胞，多核或分叶状核，似爆米花，故名爆米花样细胞（箭头所示）

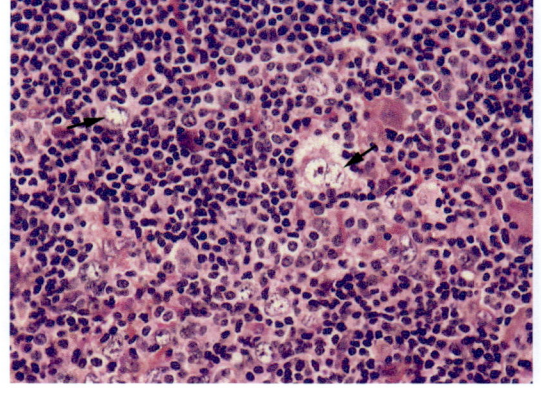

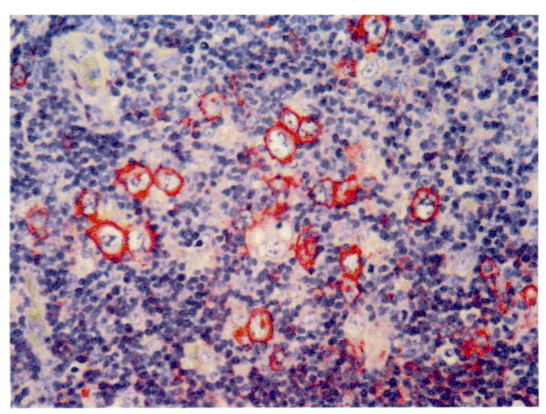

图309　结节性淋巴细胞为主型霍奇金淋巴瘤
Nodular lymphocyte predominant Hodgkin lymphoma
与图307为同一病例。免疫组化染色显示爆米花样肿瘤细胞CD20膜强阳性

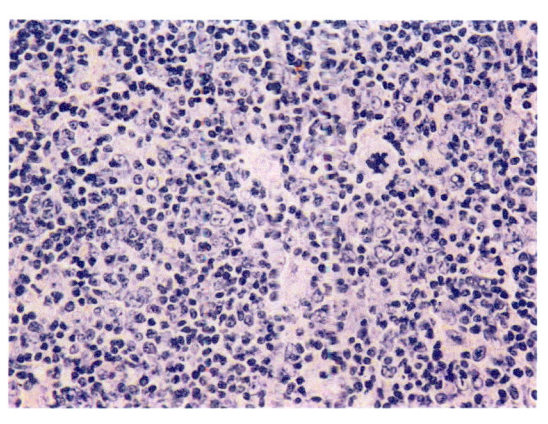

图310 结节性淋巴细胞为主型霍奇金淋巴瘤
Nodular lymphocyte predominant Hodgkin lymphoma
与图307为同一病例。免疫组化显示爆米花样肿瘤细胞CD30及CD-5均阴性

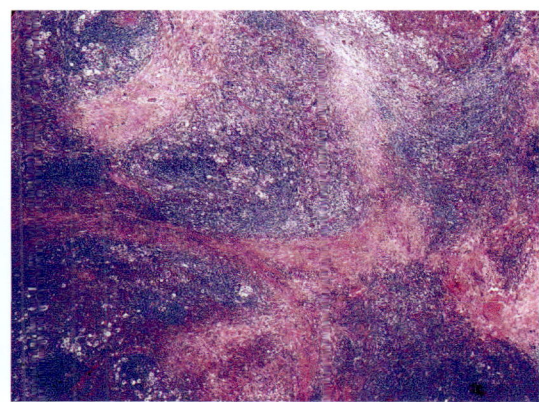

图311 经典型霍奇金淋巴瘤（结节硬化亚型）
Classical Hodgkin lymphoma (nodular sclerosis subtype)
淋巴结结构消失，代之以结节样病灶，结节周围有胶原纤维硬化带

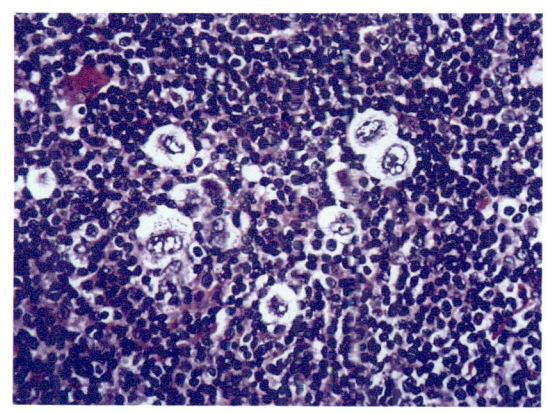

图312 经典型霍奇金淋巴瘤（结节硬化亚型）
Classical Hodgkin lymphoma (nodular sclerosis subtype)
图311高倍图。显示结节样病灶内的肿瘤细胞。其体积大，单核，胞质丰富、浅染。整个细胞似位于陷窝中，故名陷窝细胞

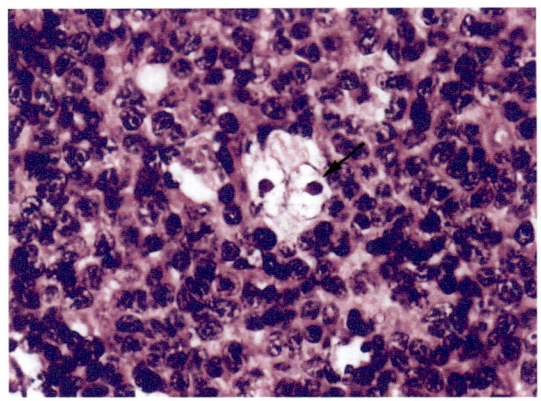

图313 经典型霍奇金淋巴瘤（混合细胞亚型）
Classical Hodgkin lymphoma (mixed cellularity subtype)
图示典型的双核R-S细胞（箭头）。瘤细胞体积大，双核、核仁大红染，两核相对排列、互为镜影，故名镜影细胞

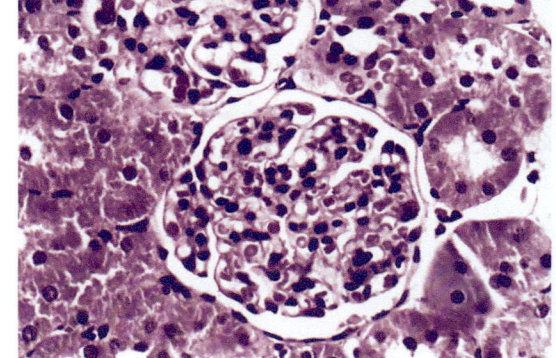

图314 正常肾小球
Normal glomerulus
肾小球由血管球和肾球囊构成，肾小球和与之相连的肾小管构成肾单位，是肾脏的基本单位

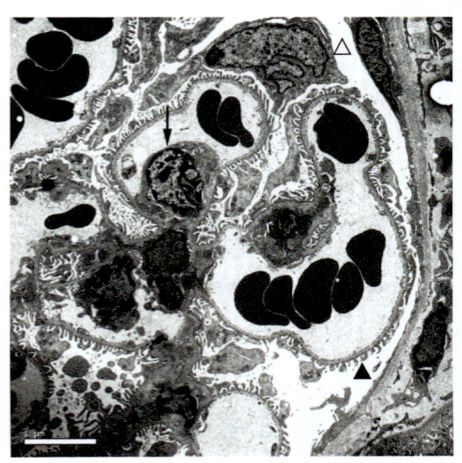

图315 正常肾小球（电镜）
Ultrastructure of normal glomerulus
肾小球的滤过膜由内皮细胞（↑）、基膜（▲）和脏层上皮细胞（△）构成

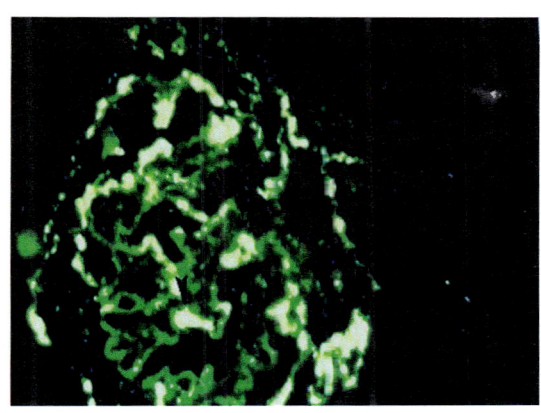

图316 免疫复合物沉积
（免疫荧光）
Deposition of immune complexes
(immunofluorescence)
IgG沿毛细血管壁呈不连续的细颗粒状、团块状沉积

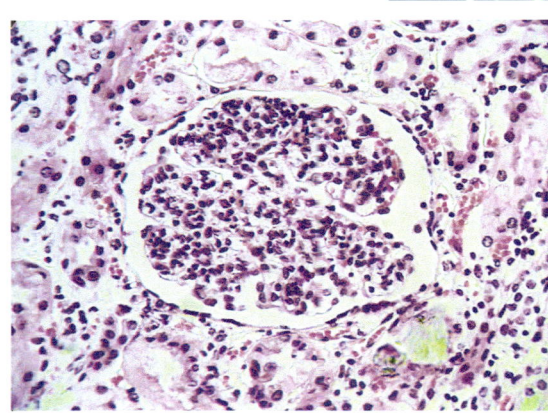

图317 急性弥漫性增生性肾小球肾炎
Acute diffuse proliferative glomerulonephritis
毛细血管内皮细胞和系膜细胞弥漫性增生，伴中性粒细胞和巨噬细胞浸润。肾小球细胞数量增多，毛细血管管腔狭窄

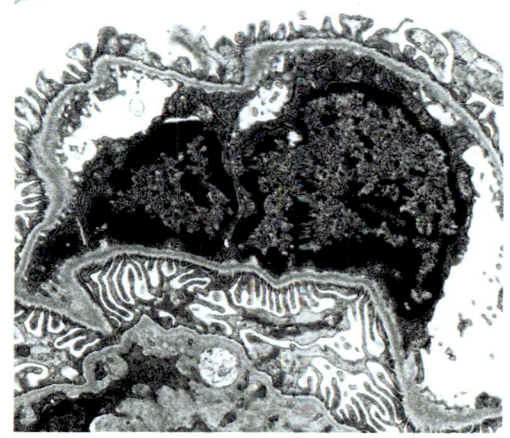

图318 急性弥漫性增生性肾小球肾炎（电镜）
Ultrastructure of acute diffuse proliferative glomerulonephritis
示内皮细胞增生肿胀

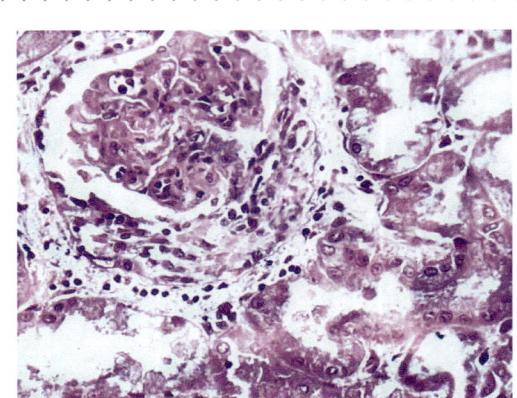

图319 新月体性肾小球肾炎
Crescentic glomerulonephritis,CrGN
肾小囊壁层上皮细胞增生，炎细胞渗出，向腔内突出，在毛细血管球外侧形成新月形结构

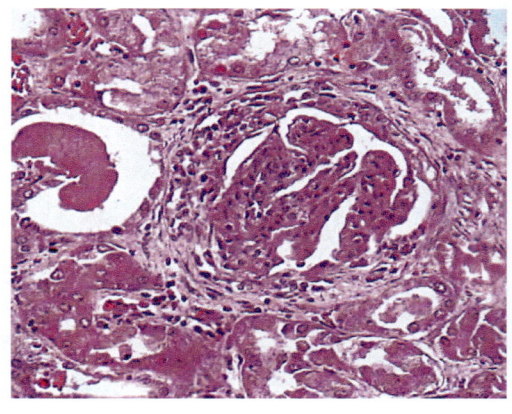

图320 新月体性肾小球肾炎（环形小体）
Crescentic glomerulonephritis,CrGN
肾小囊壁层上皮细胞弥漫增生，炎细胞渗出，在毛细血管球外侧形成环形结构

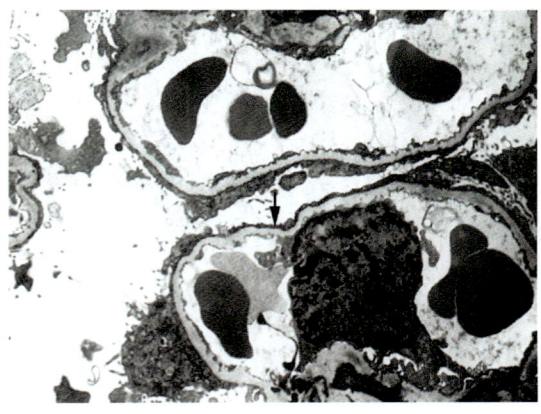

图321 轻微病变性肾小球肾炎
（电镜）
Ultrastructure of minimal change glomerulonephritis
上皮细胞变性，足突消失（↑）

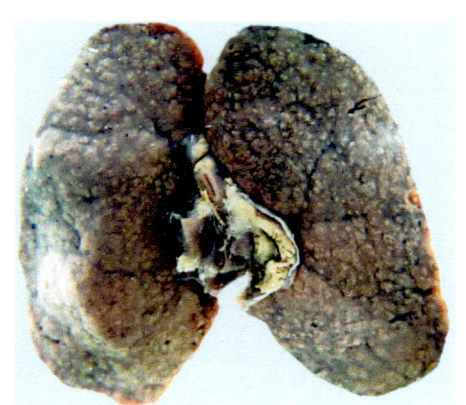

图 322 继发性颗粒性固缩肾
Secondary granular atrophy of kidney
慢性肾小球肾炎时双侧肾脏体积缩小，表面呈弥漫细颗粒状

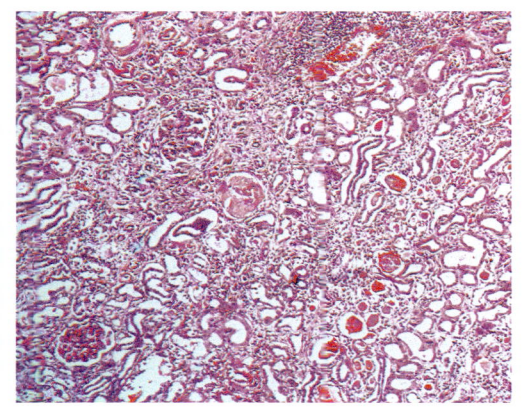

图 323 慢性肾小球肾炎
Chronic glomerulonephritis
部分肾小球萎缩、坏死、纤维化和玻璃样变，所属肾小管萎缩消失，间质可见炎性细胞浸润。部分肾小球出现代偿性增大，肾小管扩张，可见各种管型

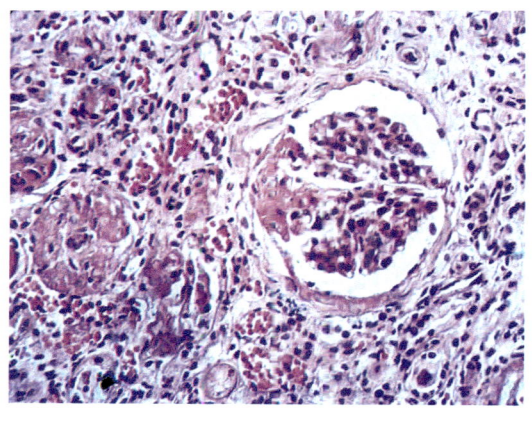

图 324 慢性肾小球肾炎
Chronic glomerulonephritis
肾小球玻璃样变和硬化，所属肾小管萎缩消失，另一肾小球部分与囊壁粘连

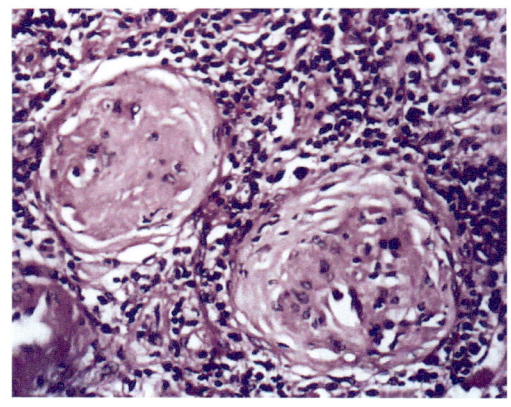

图 325　慢性肾小球肾炎
Chronic glomerulonephritis
毛细血管闭塞，肾小球玻璃样变和硬化，
所属肾小管萎缩消失

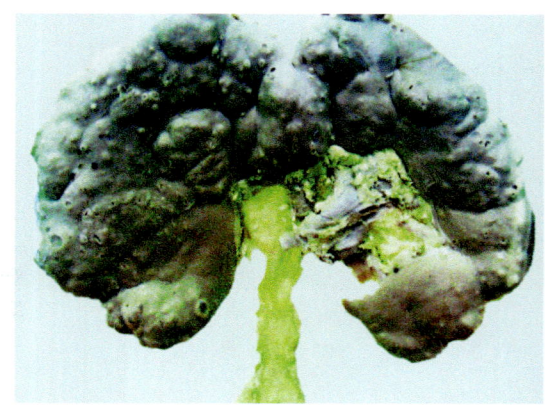

图 326　慢性肾盂肾炎
Chronic pyelonephritis
肾脏体积缩小、变形，表面颗粒状，
有不规则的瘢痕

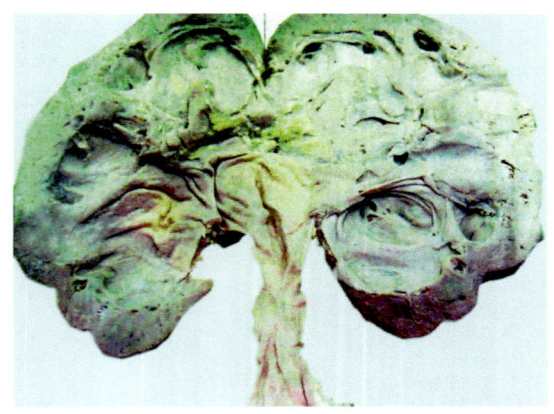

图 327　慢性肾盂肾炎
Chronic pyelonephritis
切面肾盂肾盏扩张，黏膜增厚粗糙，
肾实质受压变薄，皮髓质界线不清，
输尿管明显增粗

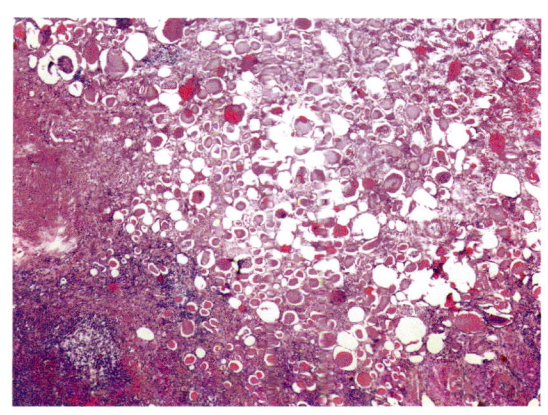

图 328 慢性肾盂肾炎
Chronic pyelonephritis
间质纤维化和炎细胞浸润,部分肾小管萎缩,部分扩张,扩张的肾小管内可出现均质红染的胶样管型,形态与甲状腺滤泡相似

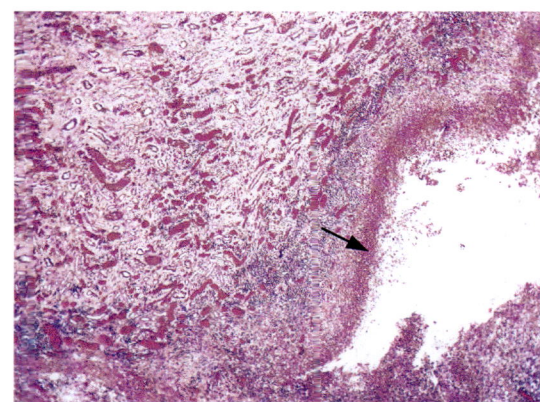

图 329 慢性肾盂肾炎急性发作
Acute paroxysm of chronic pyelonephritis
肾间质纤维化,肾小管萎缩,组织中可见一局限性脓肿灶(↑)

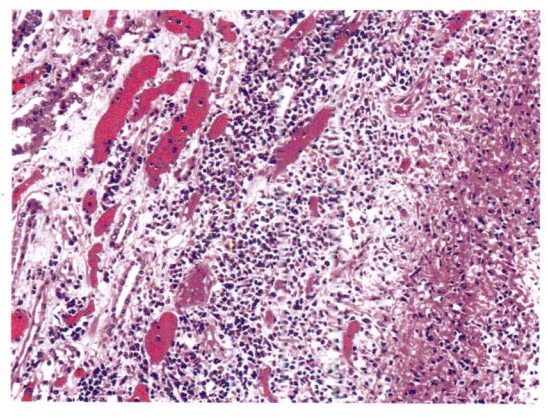

图 330 慢性肾盂肾炎急性发作
Acute paroxysm of chronic pyelonephritis
图329高倍镜下示脓肿灶周边大量毛细血管扩张及渗出的中性粒细胞

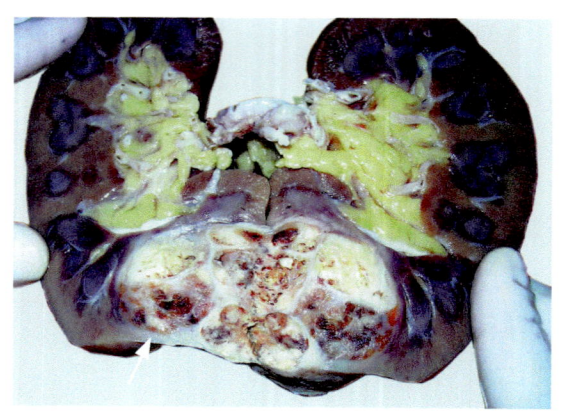

图331 肾细胞癌
Renal cell carcinoma
肾脏下极实性圆形肿物（↑），界限较清，切面淡黄色、灰白色，伴灶状出血、坏死，多种颜色交错呈多彩状

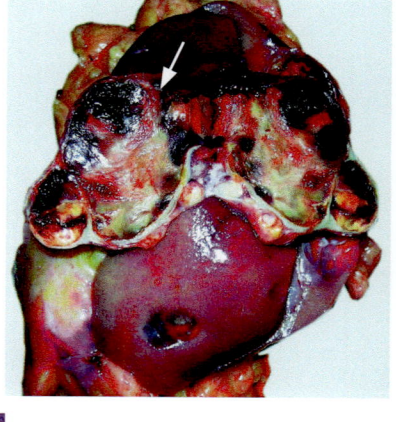

图332 肾细胞癌
Renal cell carcinoma
肾脏上中极肿物（↑），界限较清，切面呈多彩状，伴有明显的出血坏死

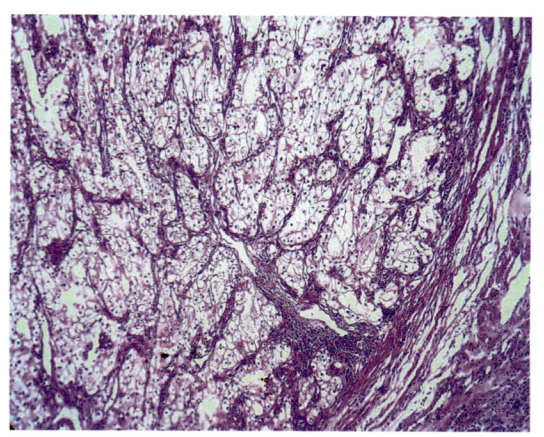

图333 肾透明细胞癌
Clear cell renal carcinoma
癌细胞呈巢片状排列，细胞大，多角形，轮廓清楚，胞浆清亮透明。核小，深染，圆形，位于细胞中央

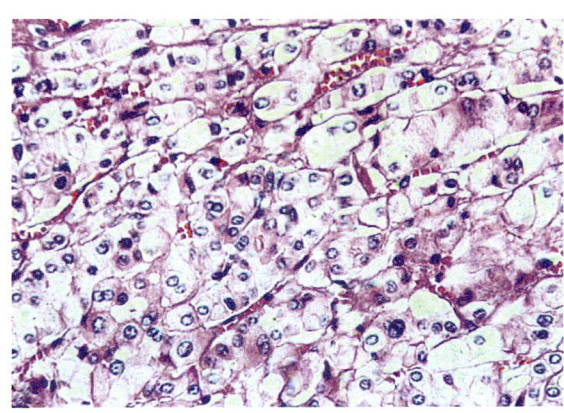

图334 肾嫌色细胞癌
Chromophobe renal carcinoma
癌细胞排列呈巢片状,细胞大小不一,胞浆淡染略嗜酸性,核大,核周常有空晕

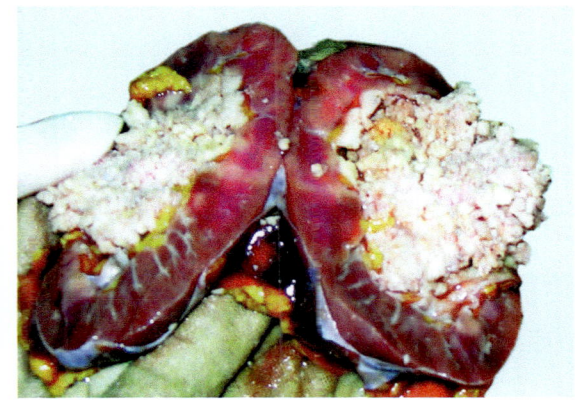

图335 肾盂移行细胞癌
Transitional cell carcinoma of renal pelvis
肾盂黏膜发生的移行细胞癌,呈外生菜花状,灰白色,填满肾盂

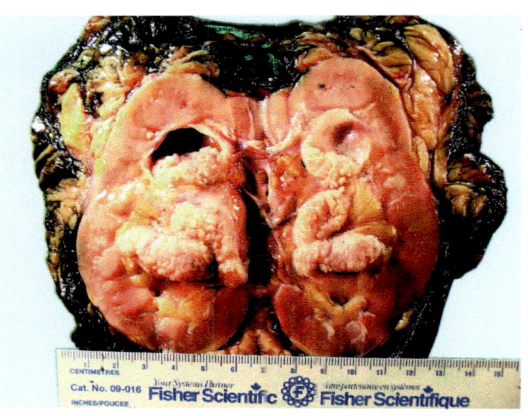

图336 肾盂移行细胞癌
Transitional cell carcinoma of renal pelvis
来源于肾盂黏膜的恶性肿瘤,呈外生性生长,堵满肾盂

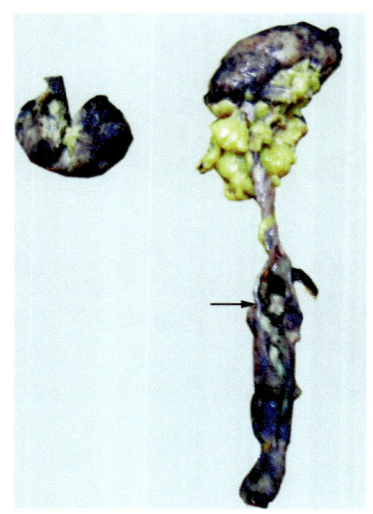

图337 输尿管移行细胞癌
Transitional cell carcinoma of ureter
输尿管中下段扩张，其内可见一外生菜花样肿物阻塞管腔（↑），上端肾脏可见压迫性萎缩

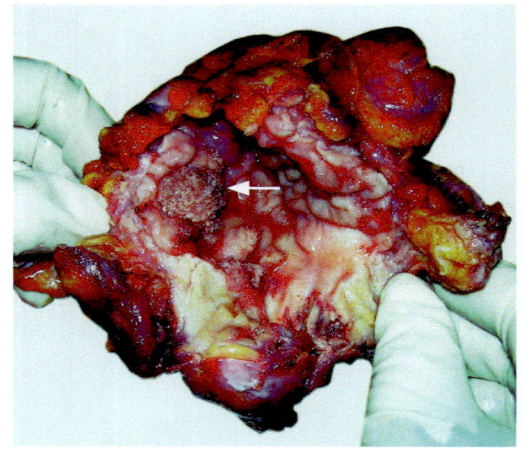

图338 膀胱癌
Carcinoma of bladder
膀胱三角区可见外生菜花样肿物（↑），灰白色，质硬，底宽无蒂，膀胱壁代偿性增厚

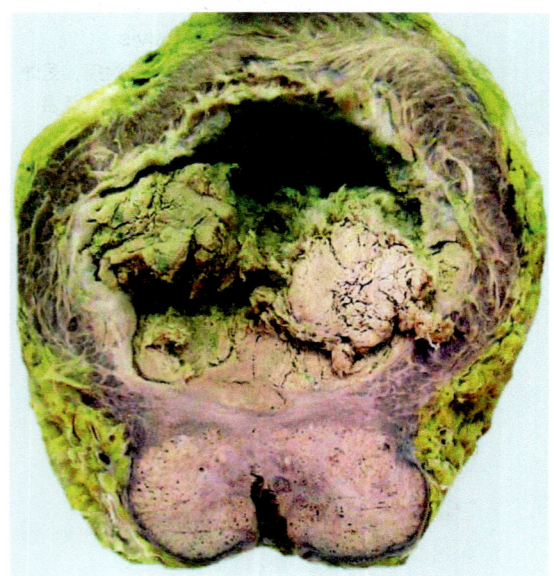

图339 膀胱癌
Carcinoma of bladder
膀胱腔内可见一外生菜花样肿物，灰白色，质硬，底宽无蒂，膀胱壁代偿性增厚

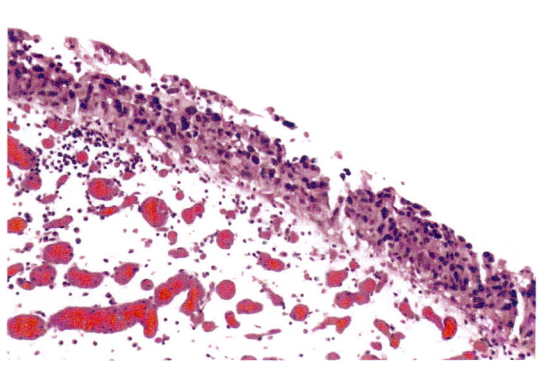

图340 膀胱移行细胞原位癌
Transitional cell carcinoma in situ of bladder
移行上皮细胞层次增多，细胞具有一定异型性，基底膜完整

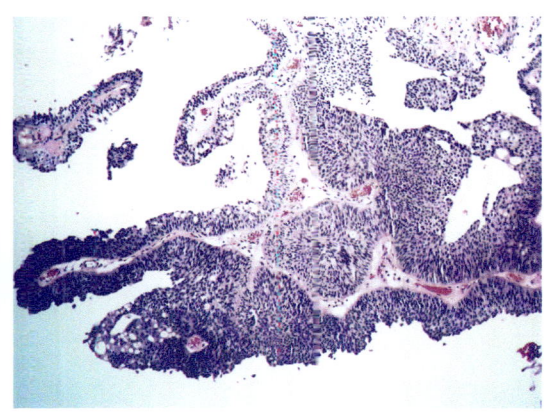

图341 膀胱乳头状移行上皮细胞癌
Papillary transitional cell carcinoma of bladder
肿瘤呈乳头状生长，乳头中轴为纤维结缔组织间质，表面被覆增生的移形上皮细胞

图342 膀胱乳头状移行上皮细胞癌
Papillary transitional cell carcinoma of bladder
增生的移形上皮细胞层次增多，缺乏从底层到表层由柱状细胞到扁平细胞逐渐分化的现象，核大小不一，间质中有丰富的毛细血管

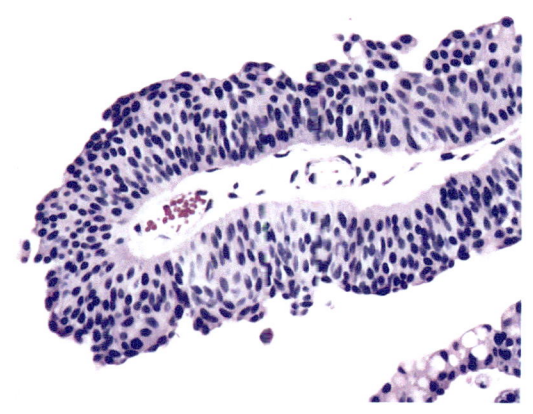

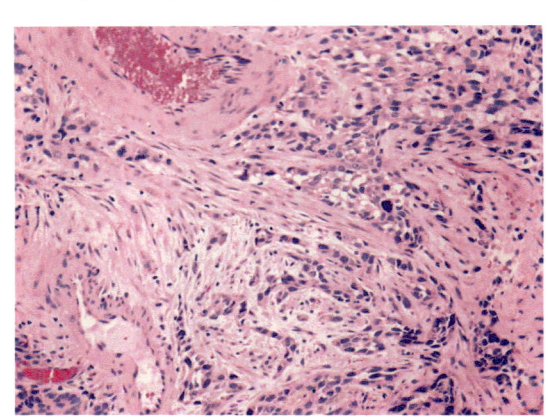

图343 膀胱浸润性移行细胞癌
Invasive transitional cell carcinoma of bladder
乳头结构不明显，细胞排列呈条索状，细胞分化差，异型性明显

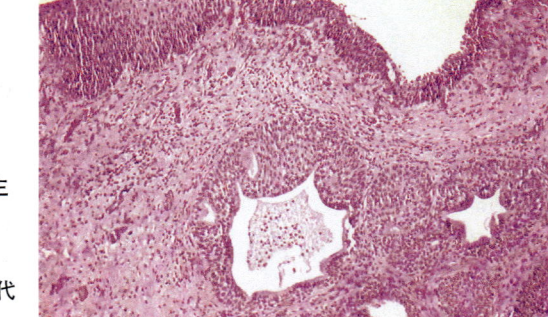

图344 膀胱炎伴鳞状上皮化生
Cystitis with squamous metaplasia
膀胱黏膜移行上皮被鳞状上皮所取代

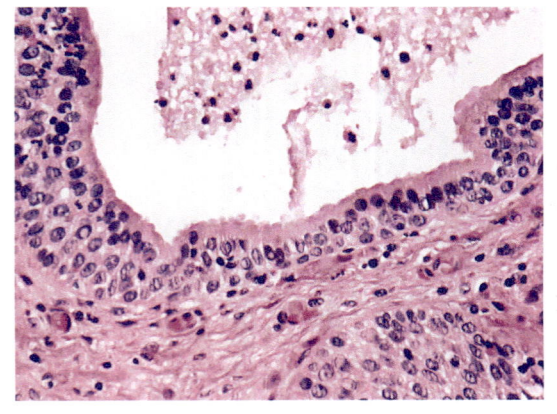

图345 膀胱炎伴鳞状上皮化生
Cystitis with squamous metaplasia
图344高倍图。示鳞状上皮化生

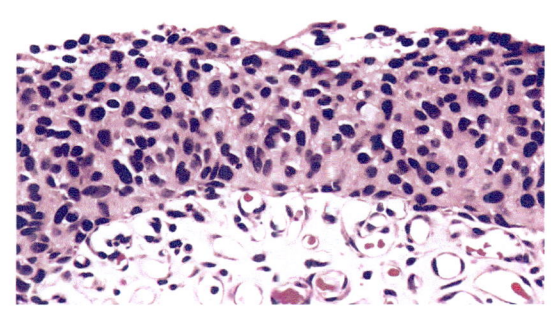

图346 膀胱鳞癌原位癌
Squamous cell carcinoma in situ of bladder
由伴鳞状上皮化生的慢性膀胱炎发展而来，细胞异型性明显，但肿瘤细胞未突破基底膜

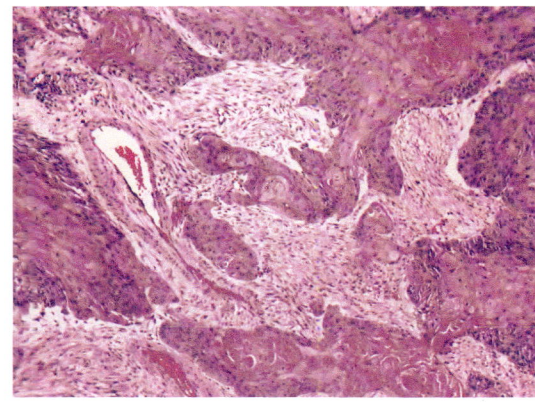

图347 膀胱高分化鳞癌
Well differentiated squamous cell carcinoma of bladder
癌细胞肌层浸润呈巢索状排列，细胞分化差，可见角化珠

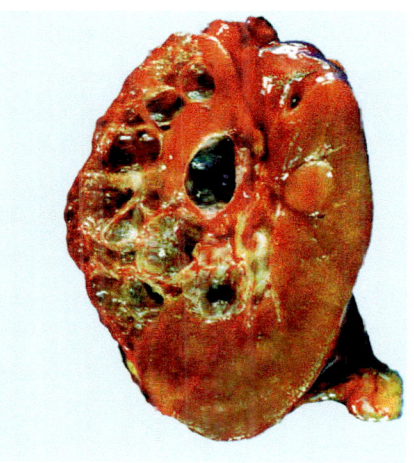

图348 多囊肾
Polycystic kidney
肾脏明显肿大，肾内遍布大小不等的囊腔，肾实质减少

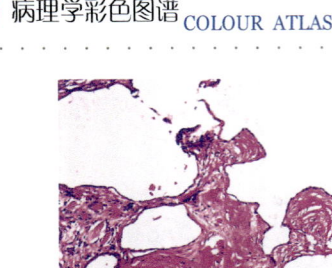

图 349　多囊肾
Polycystic kidney
光镜下可见囊壁被覆扁平上皮，可见灶状的乳头状增生。囊腔之间为残留的肾实质

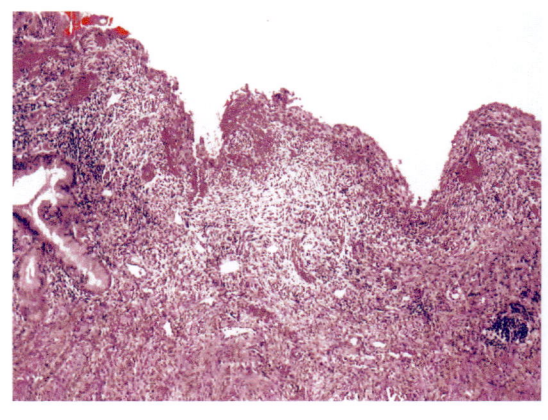

图 350　慢性宫颈炎
Chronic cervicitis
子宫颈黏膜充血水肿，间质内有淋巴细胞、浆细胞和单核细胞等慢性炎细胞浸润

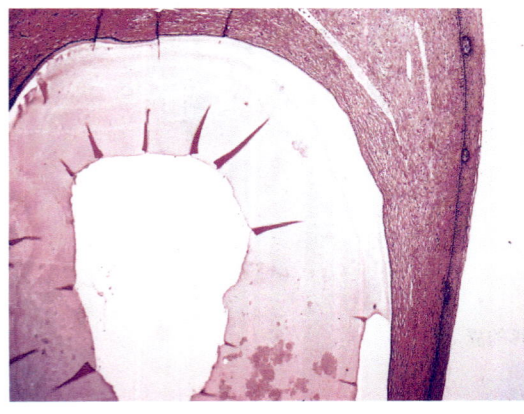

图 351　子宫颈囊肿
Nabothian cyst
又称纳博特囊肿，子宫颈腺体扩张呈囊状，囊壁被覆立方上皮，囊内含黏液

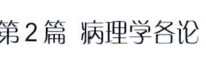

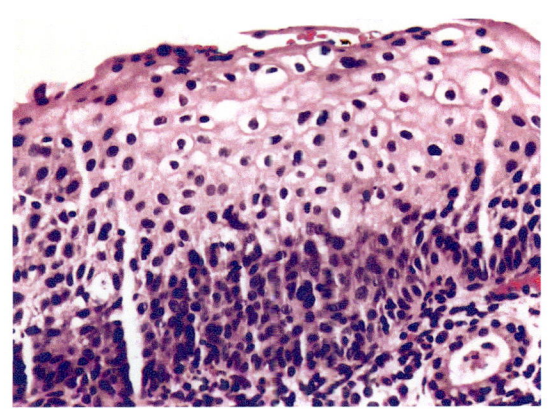

图352 子宫颈上皮内瘤变Ⅰ级
Cervical intraepithelial neoplasia, CIN Ⅰ
子宫颈上皮层内出现异型细胞,异型细胞局限于上皮层的下1/3区域

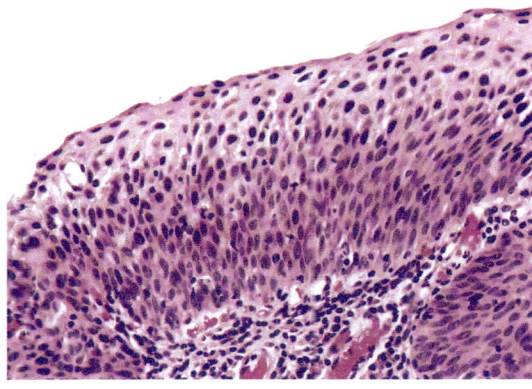

图353 子宫颈上皮内瘤变Ⅱ级
Cervical intraepithelial neoplasia, CIN Ⅱ
子宫颈上皮层内出现异型细胞,异型细胞占上皮层下1/2~2/3,细胞异型性明显,极性稍乱

图354 子宫颈上皮内瘤变Ⅲ级
Cervical intraepithelial neoplasia, CIN Ⅲ
子宫颈上皮层内出现异型细胞,异型细胞超过上皮层的下2/3,核异型性明显,上皮细胞层次消失,仅表层尚可见某些成熟的扁平细胞覆盖于表面

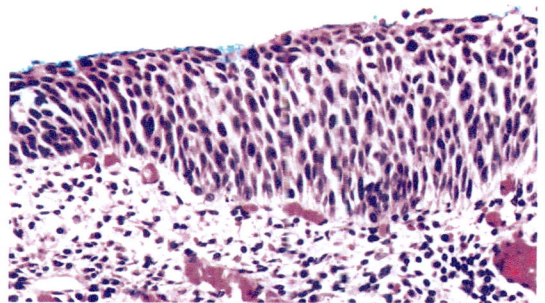

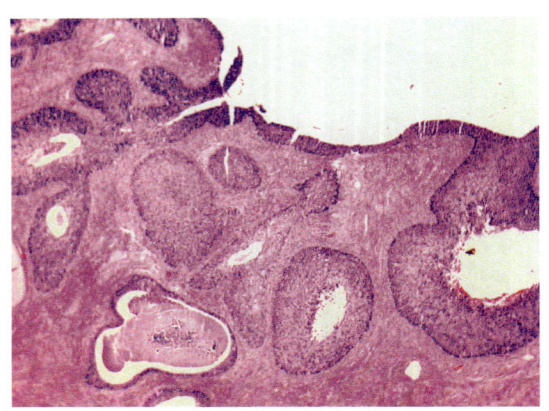

图355 子宫颈原位癌累及腺体
Carcinoma in situ of cervix and involved gland
原位癌中癌细胞沿基底膜延伸入腺体内，使整个腺体或某一部分为癌细胞所取代，但腺体轮廓尚存，腺体基底膜完整

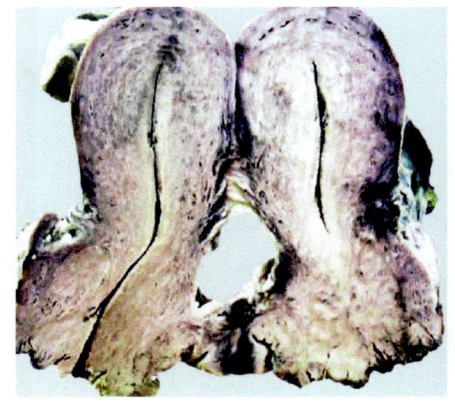

图356 子宫颈癌（内生浸润型）
Carcinoma of cervix (invasive type)
癌组织呈灰白色，向子宫颈深部浸润生长，使宫颈增大变硬

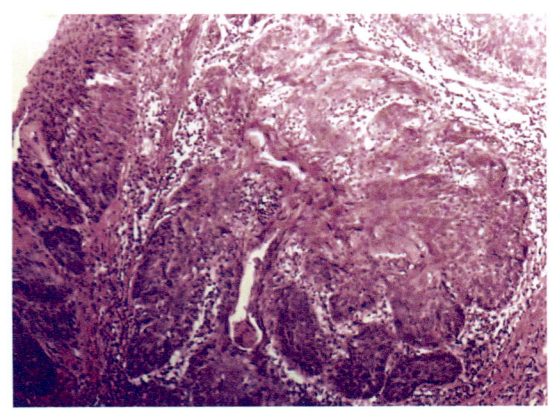

图357 子宫颈鳞状细胞癌（低分化）
Squamous cell carcinoma of cervix (poorly differentiated)
癌组织向间质内呈浸润性生长，形成团块状大小不等的癌巢

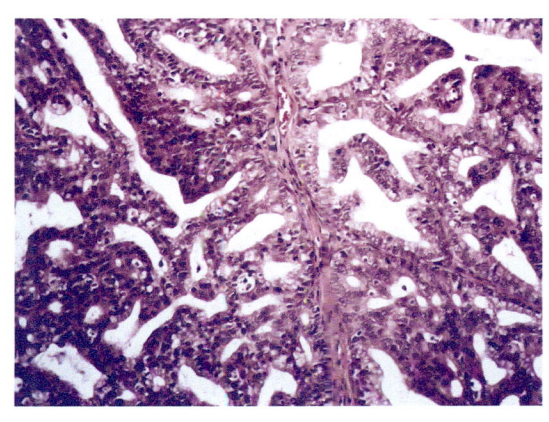

图358 子宫颈腺癌
Adenocarcinoma of cervix
癌细胞形成大小不等、形状不一、排列不规则的腺管样结构，部分腺管癌细胞增生呈复层

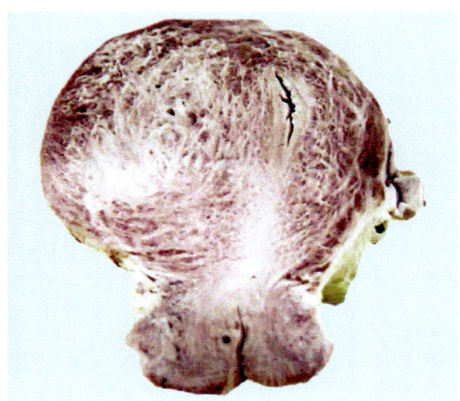

图359 子宫腺肌病
Adenomyosis of uterus
子宫内膜腺体及间质异位于子宫肌层中，子宫体增大，呈球形，切面可见散在大小不等的小腔，周围可见平滑肌纤维呈漩涡状排列

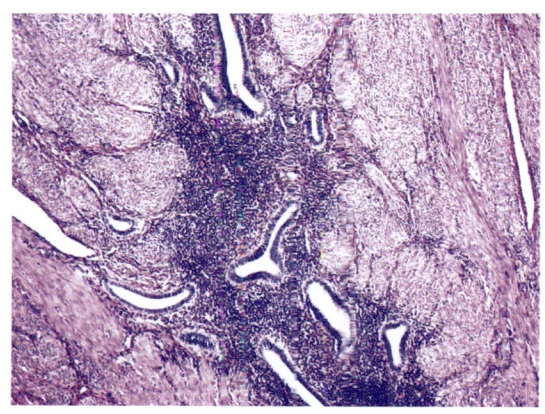

图360 子宫腺肌病
Adenomyosis of uterus
在子宫肌层中可见与正常子宫内膜相似的子宫内膜腺体、子宫内膜间质

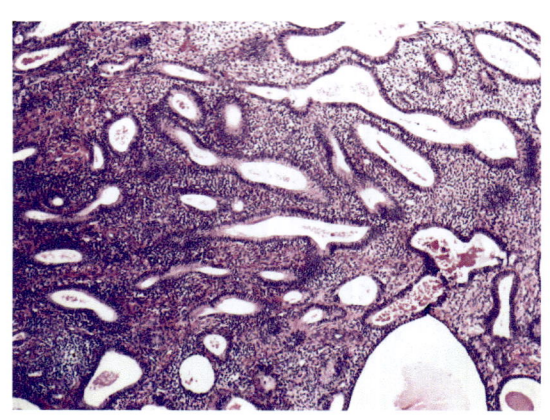

图361 子宫内膜单纯性增生
Simple hyperplasia of endometrium
腺体数量增多，结构不规则，腺上皮显示单层或假复层，无细胞异型性

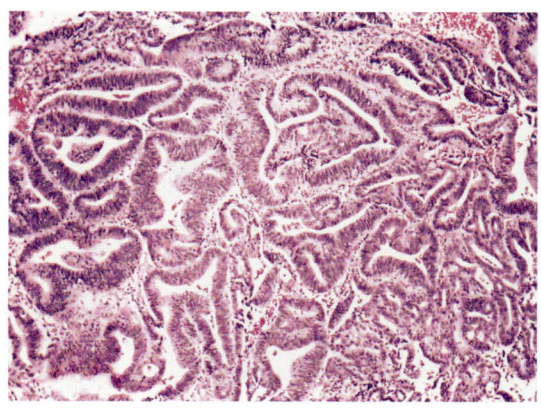

图362 子宫内膜复杂性增生
Complex hyperplasia of endometrium
腺体明显增生，结构复杂且不规则，腺上皮突向腺腔，腺体之间的间质较稀少，无细胞异型性

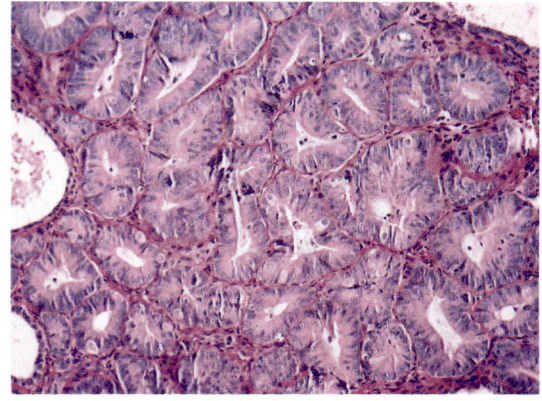

图363 子宫内膜非典型增生
Atypical hyperplasia of endometrium
子宫内膜腺体明显增生，排列拥挤，上皮细胞出现异型性，体积增大，核深染，有明显的核仁，核浆比例增大

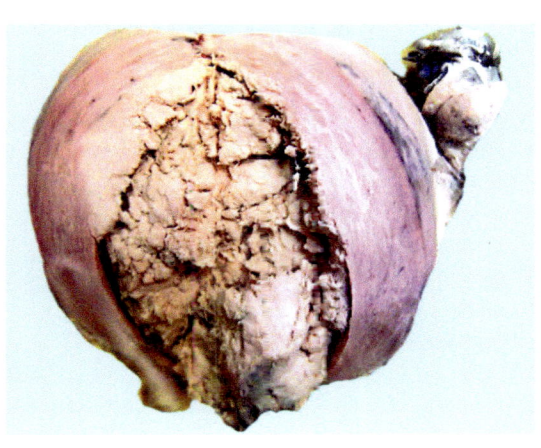

图 364 子宫内膜癌（弥漫型）
Adenocarcinoma of endometrium （diffuse type）
子宫内膜弥漫性增厚，癌组织呈灰白色，质实，充满宫腔

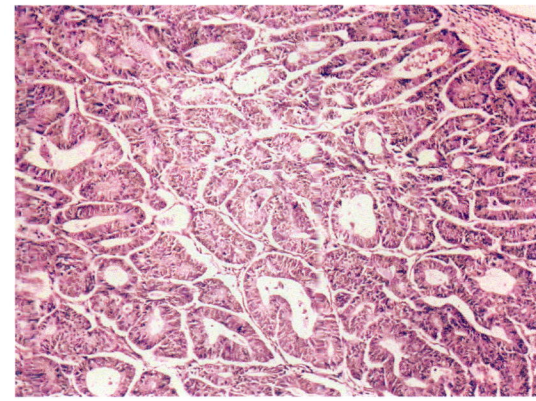

图 365 子宫内膜腺癌（高分化）
Adenocarcinoma of endometrium
（well differentiated）
癌细胞形成大小不等、形状不一腺管样结构，癌细胞轻度异型性

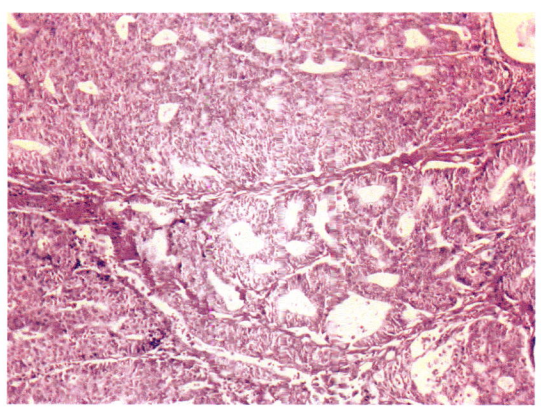

图 366 子宫内膜腺癌（中分化）
Adenocarcinoma of endometrium
（moderate differentiated）
部分癌组织形成腺管样结构，部分形成实性结构，癌细胞异型性明显，核分裂象易见

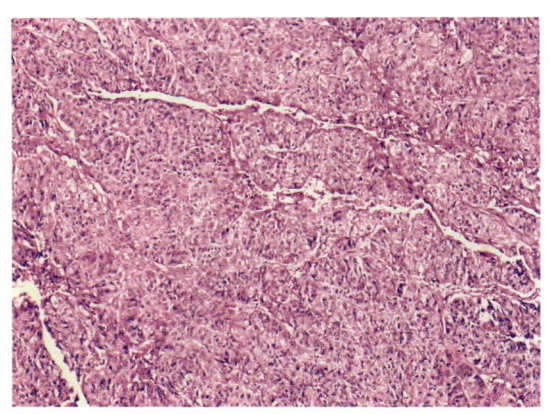

图367 子宫内膜腺癌（低分化）
Adenocarcinoma of endometrium (poorly differentiated)
大部分区域为实性片状或条索状，腺体结构很少，癌细胞异型性明显，核分裂象多见

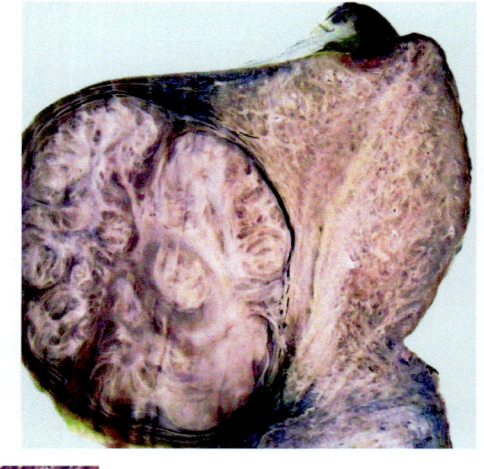

图368 子宫平滑肌瘤
Leiomyoma of uterus
肿瘤位于子宫肌层内，境界清楚，切面灰白色、编织状，挤压宫腔

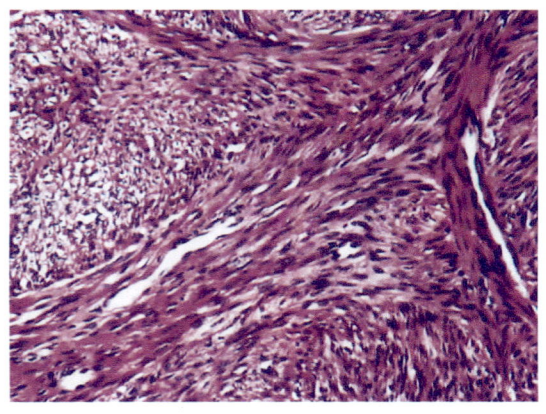

图369 子宫平滑肌瘤
Leiomyoma of uterus
瘤细胞与正常子宫平滑肌细胞相似，瘤细胞排列成束状或漩涡状

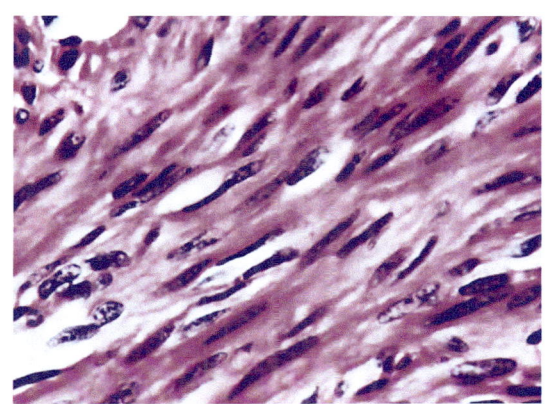

图 370 子宫平滑肌瘤
Leiomyoma of uterus
瘤细胞与正常子宫平滑肌细胞相似，梭形，胞质红染，核长杆状，两端钝圆，核分裂象少见

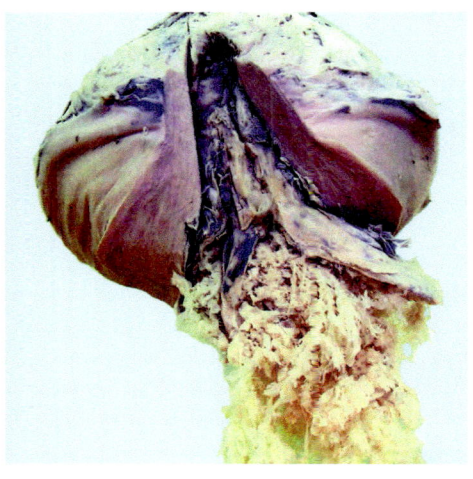

图 371 葡萄胎（完全性）
Hydatidiform mole（complete）
子宫体积增大，胎盘所有绒毛发生水肿，呈大小不等半透明的水泡状，其间有细蒂相连成串，状似葡萄

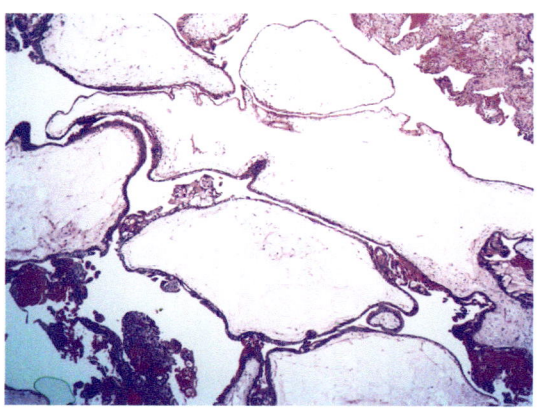

图 372 葡萄胎（完全性）
Hydatidiform mole（complete）
胎盘绒毛间质高度水肿，血管减少甚至完全消失，滋养层细胞呈不同程度的增生，并有轻度异型性

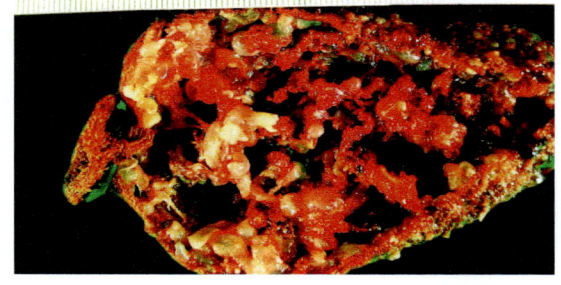

图373 葡萄胎（部分性）
Hydatidiform mole（partial）
胎盘绒毛部分发生水肿呈葡萄状，部分正常

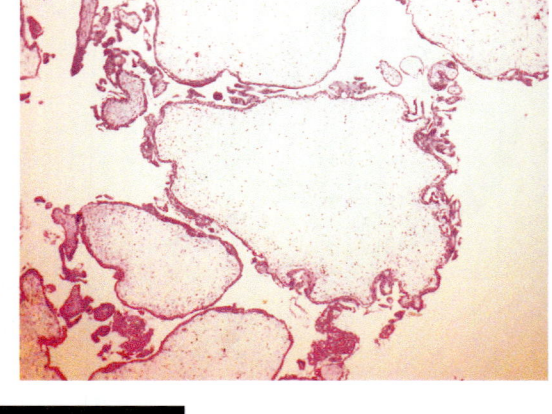

图374 葡萄胎（部分性）
Hydatidiform mole（partial）
部分胎盘绒毛高度水肿，间质血管消失，滋养层细胞呈不同程度的增生，部分正常绒毛

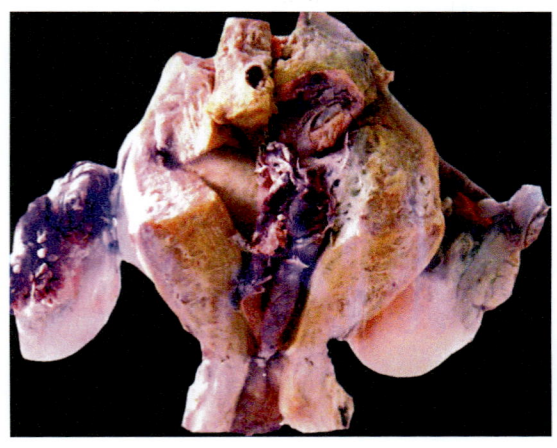

图375 侵蚀性葡萄胎
Invasive mole
水泡状绒毛侵入子宫肌层内，形成紫蓝色出血坏死结节，并穿入阔韧带内形成肿块

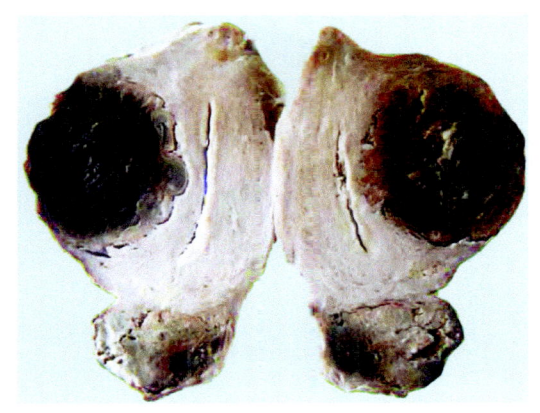

图376 子宫绒毛膜癌
Choriocarcinoma
癌组织位于子宫体部,呈紫红色,结节状,可见出血坏死,蔓延至子宫颈

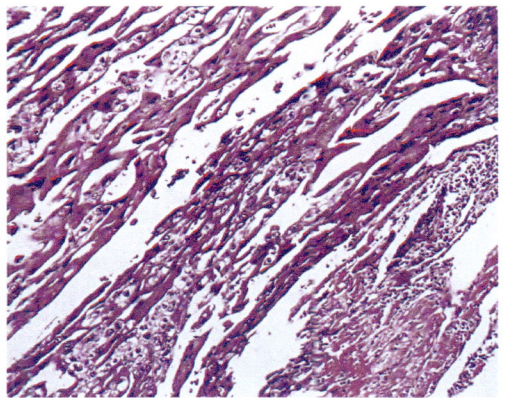

图377 子宫绒毛膜癌
Choriocarcinoma
肿瘤细胞形成索条状、片状不规则癌巢,癌组织中无间质,出血坏死明显

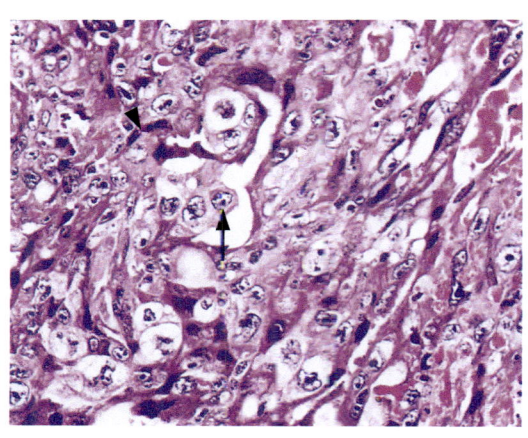

图378 子宫绒毛膜癌
Choriocarcinoma
癌组织由似细胞滋养层细胞(↑)和似合体滋养层细胞(▲)组成,细胞异型性明显

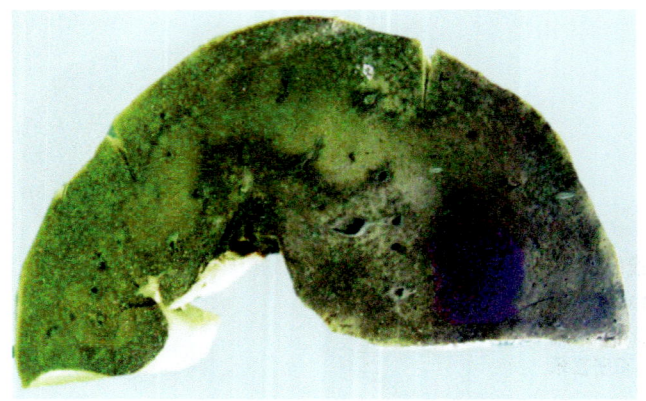

图379 子宫绒癌肝转移
Choriocarcinoma metastasis to liver
肝叶内可见一肿块，呈暗红色，质软，边界较清楚

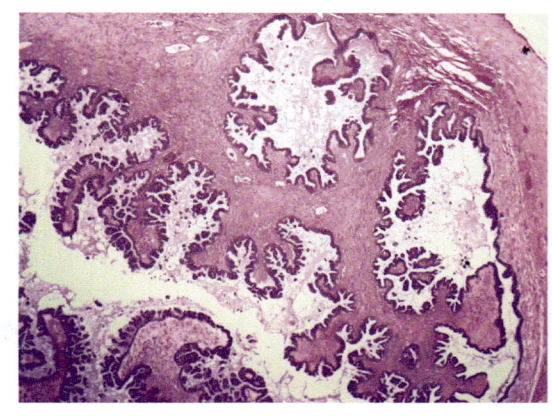

图380 卵巢交界性浆液性乳头状囊腺瘤
Borderline serous papillary cystadenoma of ovary
肿瘤呈乳头状生长，乳头上皮层次增加，达2~3层，细胞有异型性，但无间质和包膜浸润

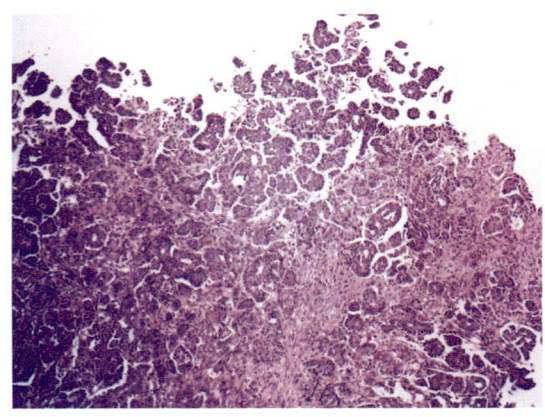

图381 卵巢浆液性乳头状囊腺癌
Serous papillary cystadenocarcinoma of ovary
瘤细胞排列紊乱，形成短分支乳头、筛状或片块状，细胞异型性明显，并向间质浸润

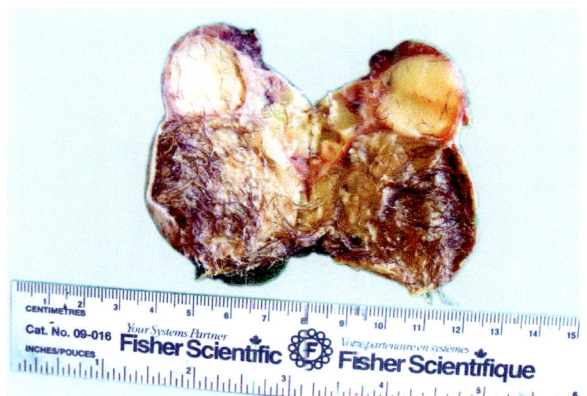

图382 卵巢成熟畸胎瘤
Mature teratoma of ovary
肿瘤呈囊性，充满皮脂样物，其中混有数量不等的毛发。囊壁上可见一个向腔内突出的实性结节，结节表面有毛发。此种类型肿瘤又称为皮样囊肿

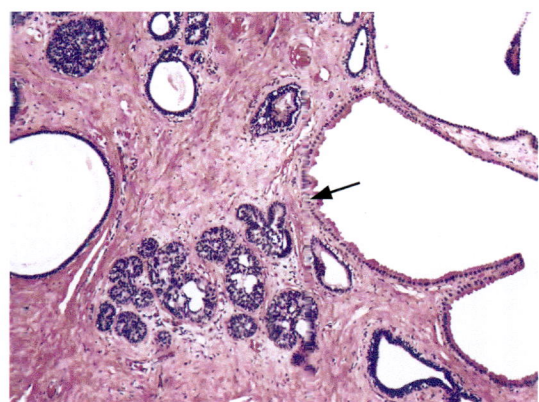

图383 乳腺增生性纤维囊性变
Hyperplasia fibrocystic change of breast
小导管扩张呈囊状，腺泡上皮增生，层次增多，局部呈筛状结构，间质纤维组织增生，并可见大汗腺化生（↑）

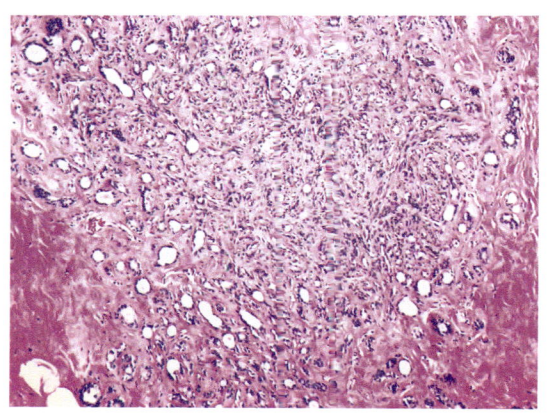

图384 乳腺硬化性腺病
Sclerosing adenosis of breast
小叶体积增大，轮廓尚存，末梢导管上皮、肌上皮和间质纤维组织增生，腺泡受压而扭曲，甚至成条索状

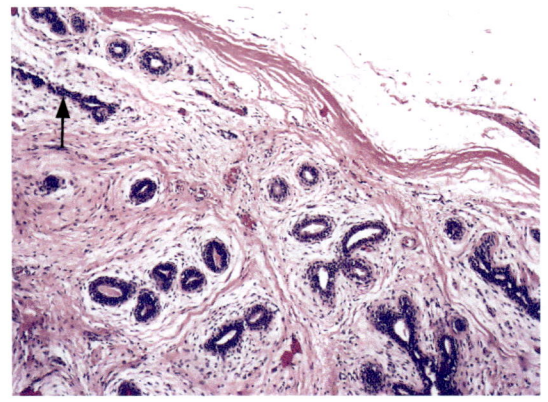

图 385 乳腺纤维腺瘤
Fibroadenoma of breast
肿瘤由增生的纤维组织和腺体组成，腺体呈圆形或卵圆形，或被增生的纤维组织挤压呈裂隙状（↑），间质较疏松，肿瘤表面有纤维被膜

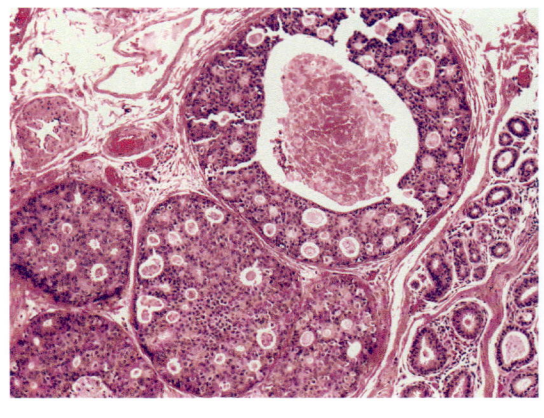

图 386 乳腺粉刺癌
Comedocarcinoma of breast
导管内癌细胞呈实性排列，中央有坏死，基底膜完整，导管周围有纤维组织增生和慢性炎细胞浸润

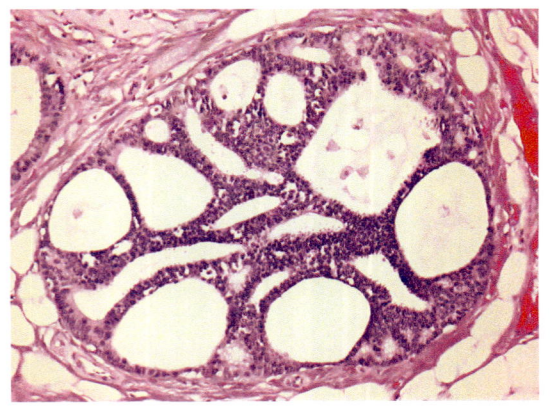

图 387 乳腺导管内原位癌
Intraductal carcinoma in situ of breast
导管内癌细胞排列成筛状，细胞体积较小，形态比较规则，基底膜完整，无坏死

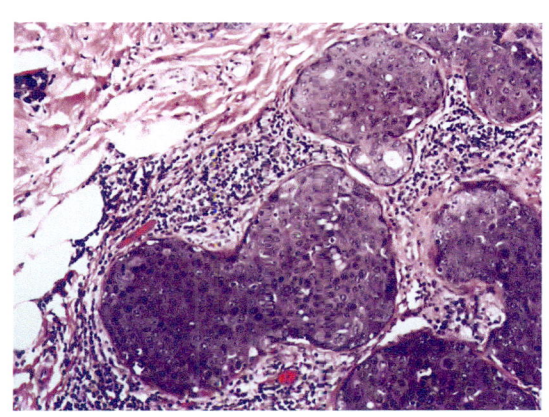

图388 乳腺导管内原位癌
Intraductal carcinoma in situ of breast
导管内癌细胞排列成实性，细胞体积较小，形态比较规则，基底膜完整，无坏死

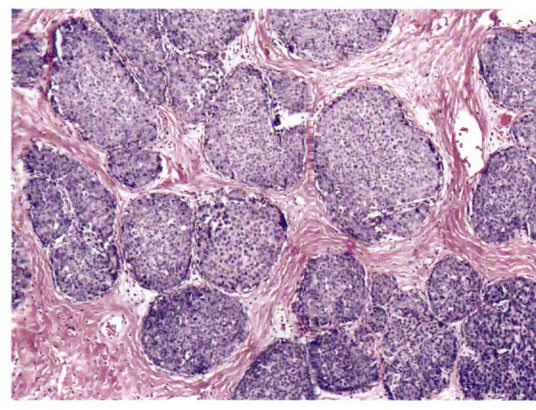

图389 乳腺小叶原位癌
Lobular carcinoma in situ of breast
乳腺小叶末梢导管和腺泡内充满呈实性排列的癌细胞，癌细胞体积小，大小形态较为一致，基底膜完整

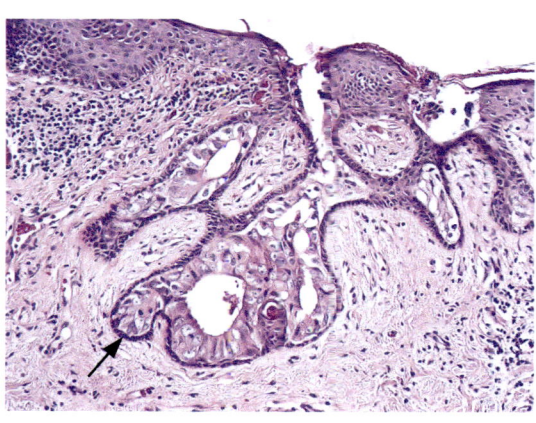

图390 乳腺Paget病
Paget's disease of breast
在乳头表皮内可见Paget细胞（↑），癌细胞体积大，胞质透明，核仁清楚，孤立散在或成簇分布

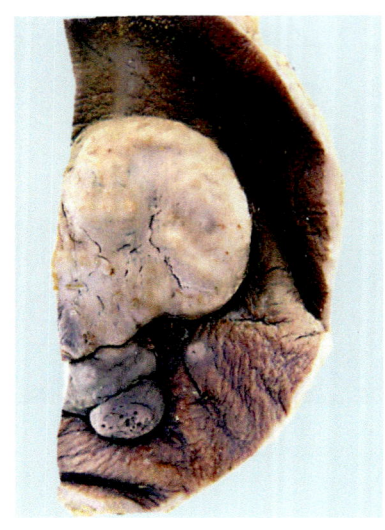

图391 乳腺癌
Carcinoma of breast
肿瘤呈灰白色，火山口状，质硬

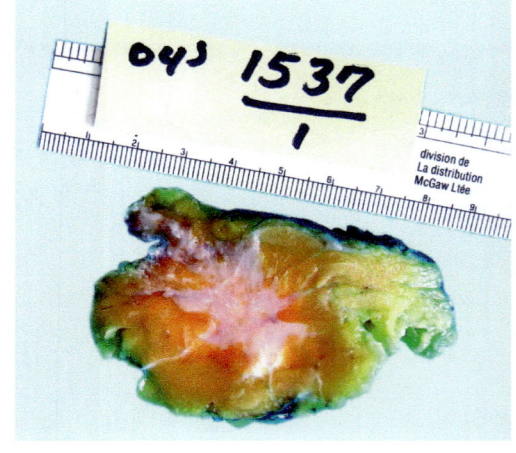

图392 乳腺癌
Carcinoma of breast
肿瘤呈灰白色，质硬，无包膜，向周围组织呈树根状浸润性生长

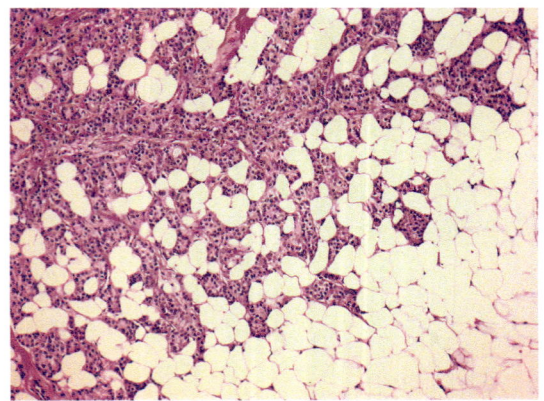

图393 乳腺浸润性导管癌
Invasive ductal carcinoma of breast
癌组织排列成巢状、索条状，呈浸润性生长

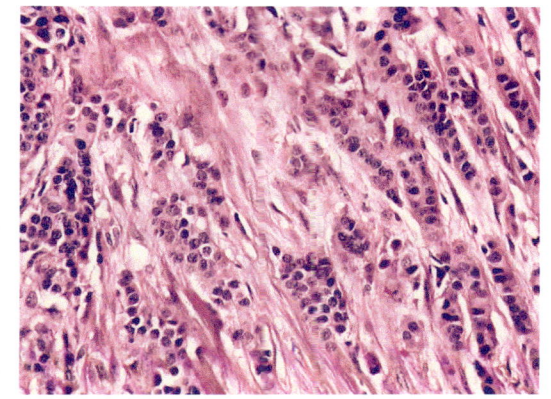

图394 乳腺浸润性导管癌（硬癌）
Invasive ductal carcinoma of breast（scirrhous carcinoma）
癌细胞排列呈索条状，细胞异型性明显，间质内有大量致密的结缔组织增生

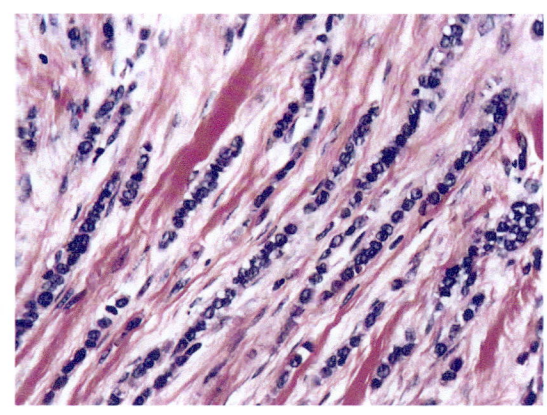

图395 乳腺浸润性小叶癌
Invasive lobular carcinoma of breast
癌细胞呈单行串珠状或细条索状浸润于纤维间质中，癌细胞体积小，大小一致，核分裂象少见

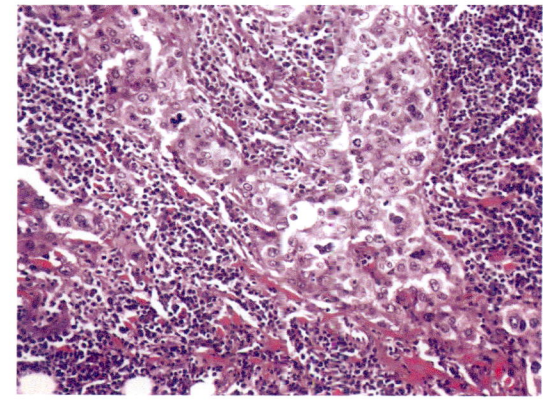

图396 乳腺髓样癌
Medullary carcinoma of breast
癌细胞体积大，呈条索、片块状排列，癌实质多，间质少，伴有丰富的淋巴细胞、浆细胞浸润

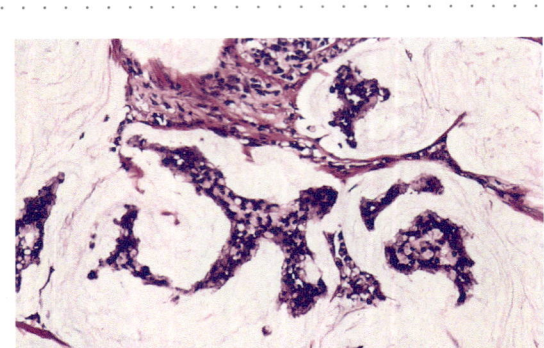

图397 乳腺黏液癌
Mucinous carcinoma of breast
癌细胞产生大量黏液，形成大片淡蓝染色的黏液湖，癌细胞聚集成小岛状，漂浮在黏液中，少数癌细胞浆内可见黏液空泡

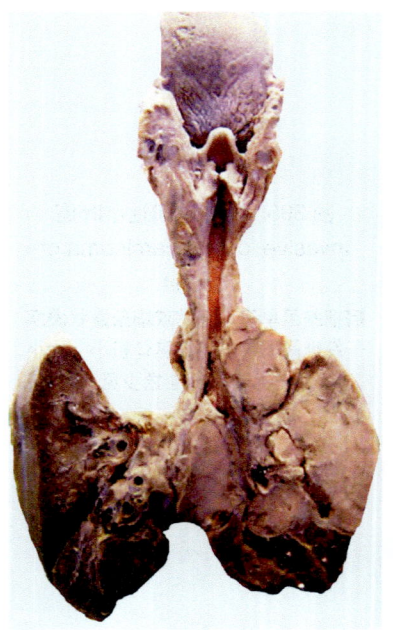

图398 原发进行性肺结核
Primary progressive pulmonary tuberculosis
肺门淋巴结肿大伴干酪样坏死，右侧肺组织可见大片结核病灶并有空洞形成；左肺呈粟粒性肺结核

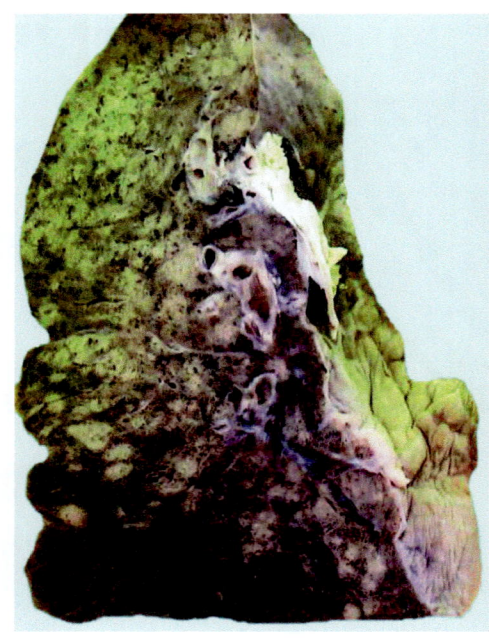

图399 干酪性肺炎
Caseous pneumonia
肺组织内可见灰黄色干酪样坏死物相互融合呈片状

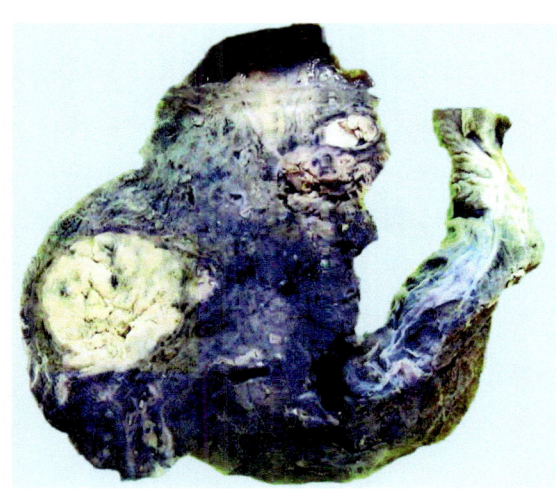

图400 肺结核球
Pulmonary tuberculoma
肺内可见一个孤立的、有纤维包裹的球形干酪样坏死物，直径约2.5cm

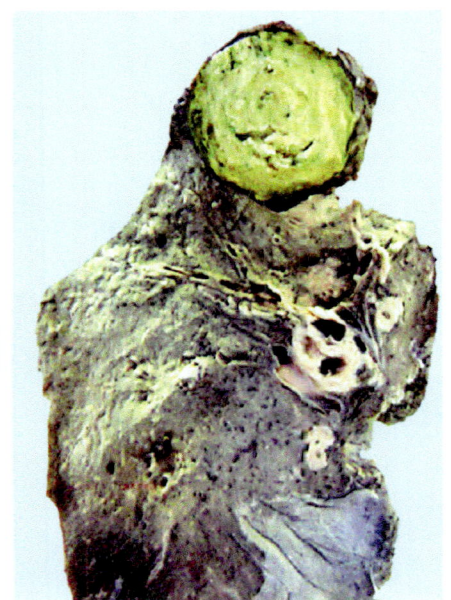

图401 肺结核球
Pulmonary tuberculoma
肺尖部可见一个孤立的、有纤维包裹的球形干酪样坏死物，直径约3cm

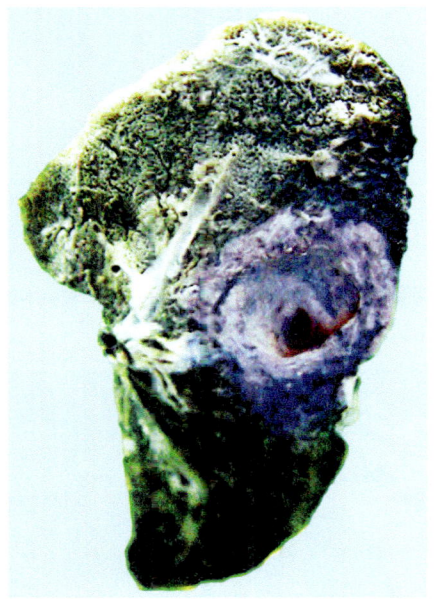

图402 慢性纤维空洞型肺结核
Chronic fibro-cavitative pulmonary tuberculosis
肺内可见一个厚壁空洞，壁厚约1.5cm

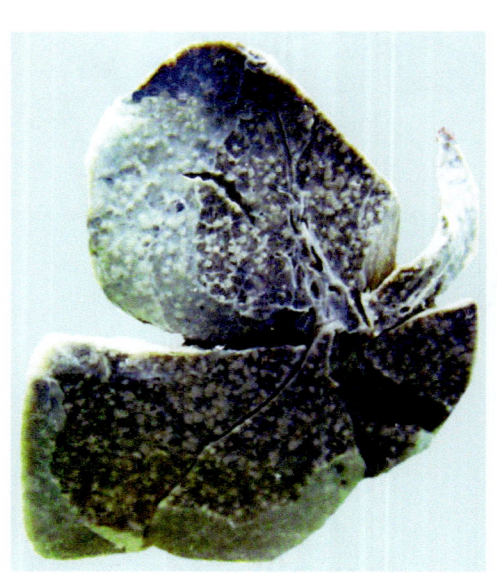

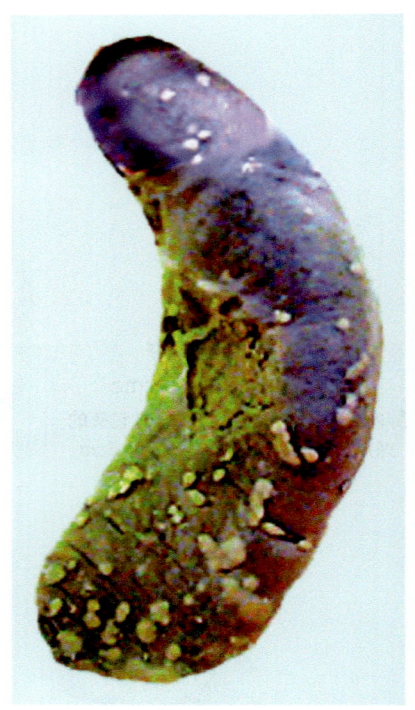

图 403　粟粒性肺结核
Miliary tuberculosis of lung
肺组织内可见大量灰白色、均匀分布的小米粒大小的病灶

图 404　脾粟粒性结核
Miliary tuberculosis of spleen
脾脏表面见均匀一致，小米粒大小，灰白色结核病灶

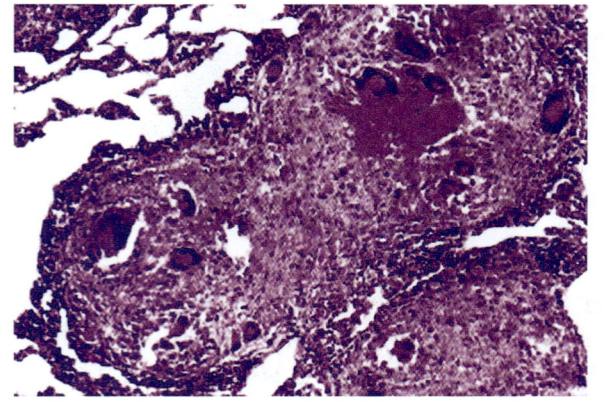

图 405　肺结核结节
Tubercle of lung
由中央干酪样坏死，周围上皮样细胞、朗格汉斯巨细胞及聚集的淋巴细胞和少量反应增生的成纤维细胞构成

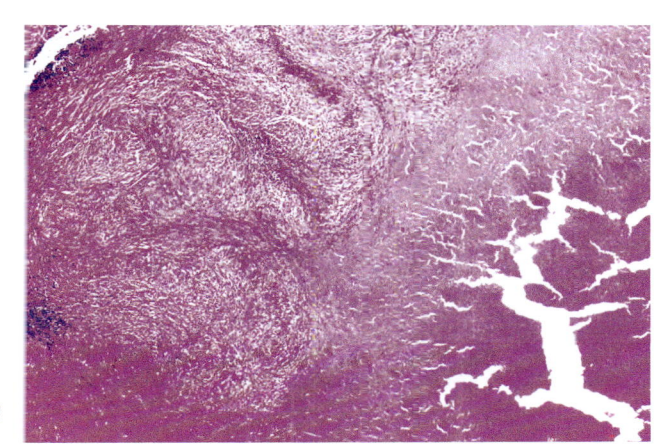

图406 结核结节
Tubercle
中心红染的干酪样坏死物

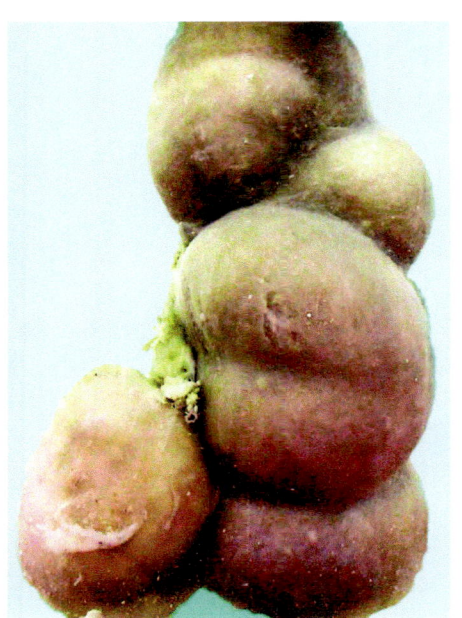

图407 淋巴结结核
Tuberculosis of lymph nodes
表面淋巴结肿大，相互粘连

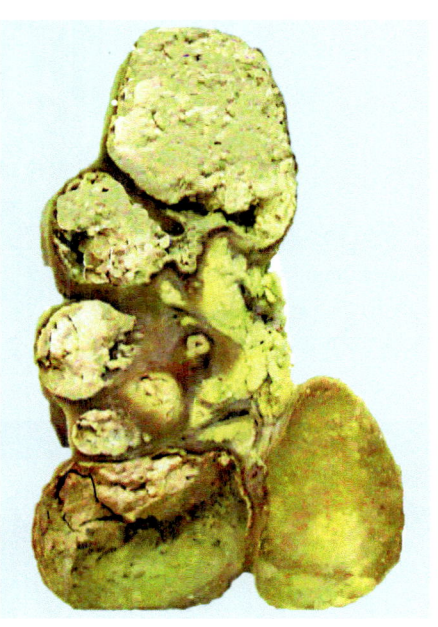

图408 淋巴结结核
Tuberculosis of lymph nodes
切面淋巴结正常结构消失，可见大量干酪样坏死物

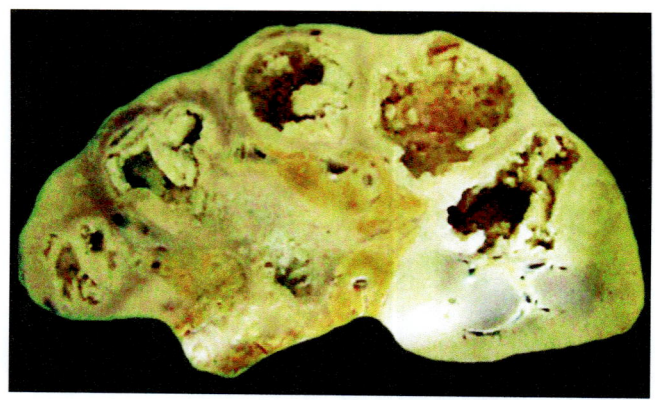

图 409 肾结核
Tuberculosis of kidney
肾切面组织结构破坏形成多个空腔，腔壁可见残存干酪样坏死物

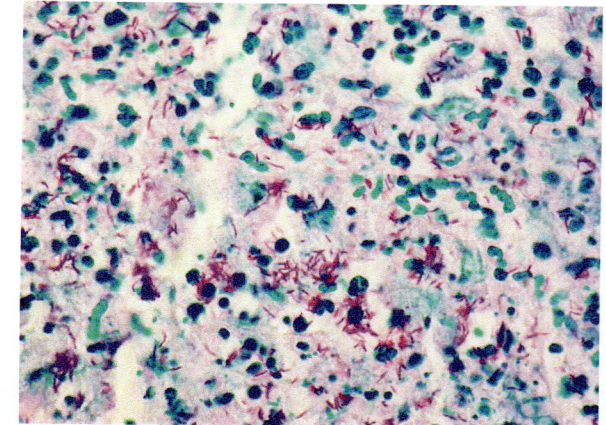

图 410 结核菌抗酸染色
Anti-acid stain of tubercle bacillus
镜下可见细小红色为结核杆菌

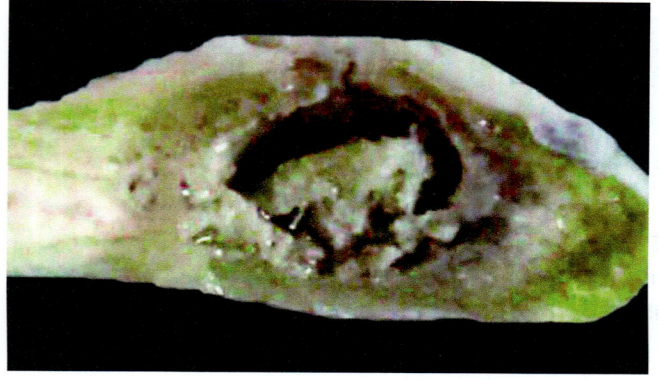

图 411 骨结核
Tuberculosis of bone
切面指骨部分结构破坏被干酪样坏死取代

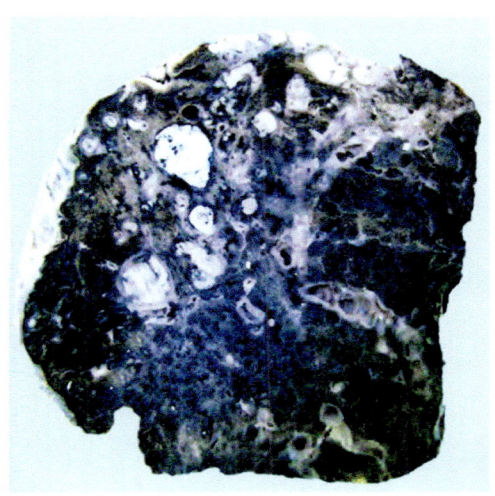

图 412 肺结核钙化灶
Calcification of pulmonary tuberculosis
肺组织切面见大小不等的瓷白色团块

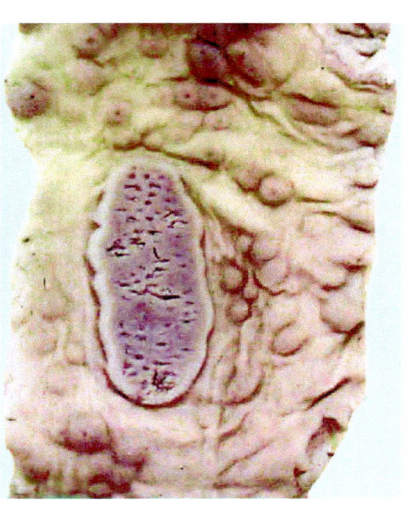

图 413 肠伤寒髓样肿胀期
Typhoid fever of intestine, stage of medullary swelling
肠壁淋巴组织肿胀，隆起于黏膜表面。以集合淋巴小结肿胀最为突出，表面形似脑回样隆起

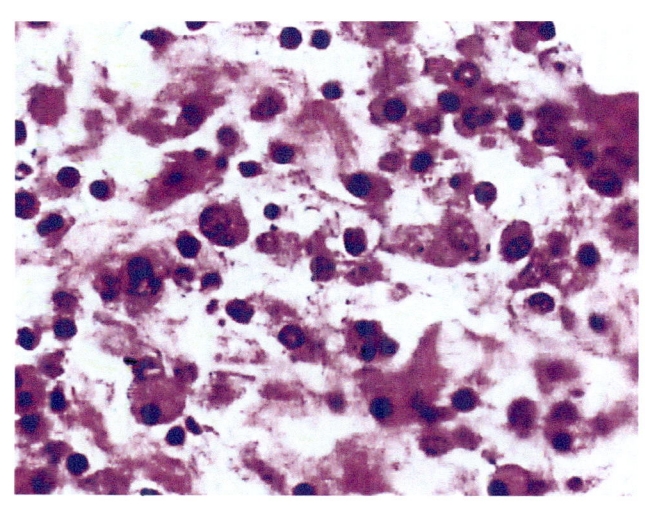

图 414 伤寒小结
Typhoid nodule
大量伤寒细胞聚集形成肉芽肿病灶

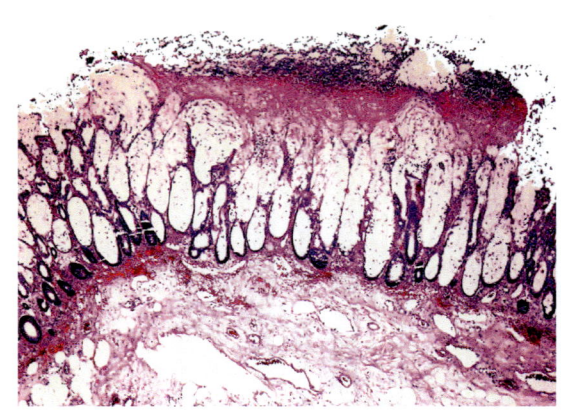

图 415　假膜性肠炎
Pseudomembrane enteritis
肠黏膜表层渗出大量红染纤维素、炎细胞，伴有肠黏膜组织坏死，共同形成假膜贴附于黏膜表面

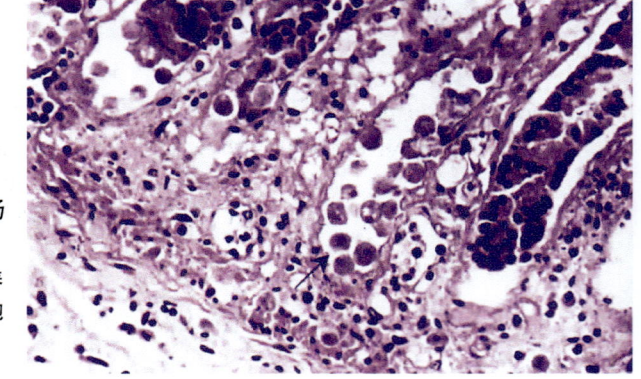

图 416　阿米巴痢疾的结肠
Amoebiasis of colon
镜下肠黏膜内可见阿米巴滋养体，圆形，巨噬细胞大小，胞浆内可见吞噬物

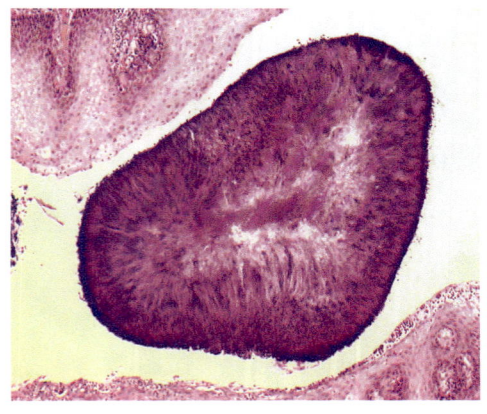

图 417　扁桃体放线菌
Tonsil actinomycete
病灶中的"硫磺颗粒"，周围部分菌丝排列成放线状；菌丝末端膨大呈棒状

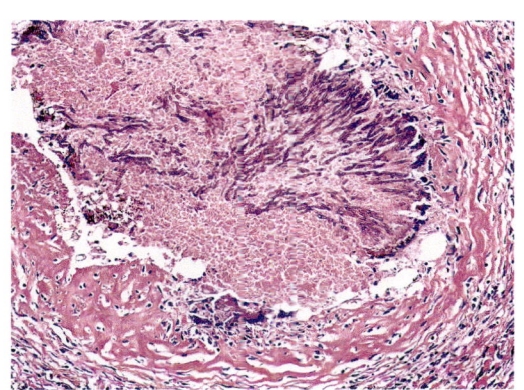

图 418 曲菌感染（PAS 染色）
Aspergillus infection（PAS stain）
曲菌红染，菌丝粗细均匀，有隔，呈锐角分枝

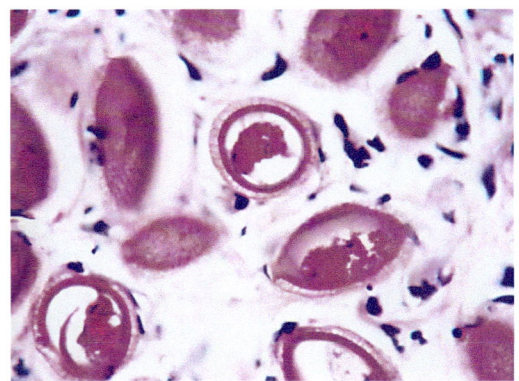

图 419 血吸虫虫卵
Eggs of schitosoma

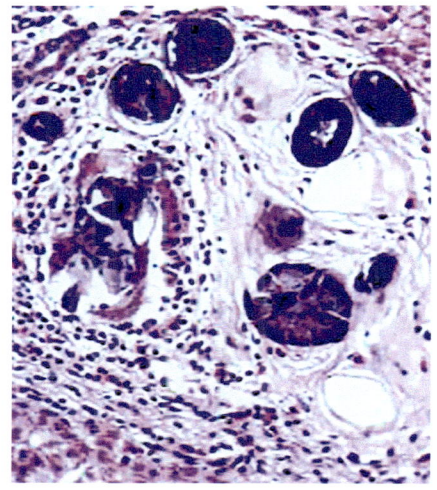

图 420 血吸虫病慢性虫卵结节
Chronic egg tubercle of schistosomiasis
结节中央有多个破裂和钙化的虫卵，形成假结核结节

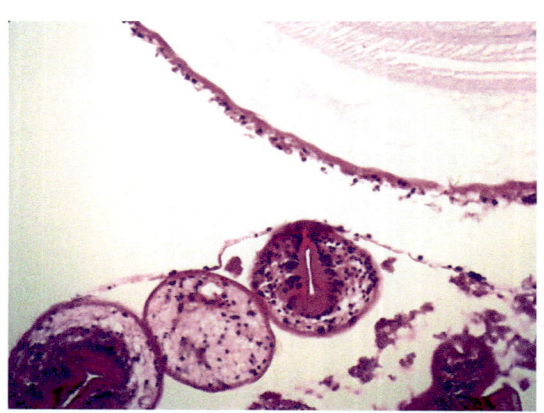

图421　细粒棘球蚴病
Echinococosis
图中可见棘球蚴（包囊虫），囊壁有内外两层，外层为纤维包膜，内囊为虫体本身。镜下红染平行板层结构为内囊的外层，内层为生发层，由生发细胞构成

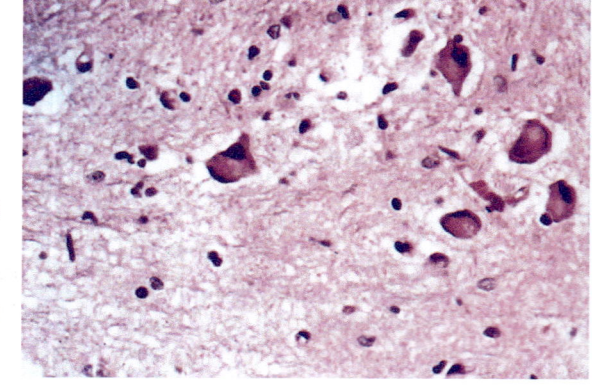

图422　乙脑时嗜神经细胞象
Epidemic encephalitis B,
engulfing nerve cells
退变的神经细胞胞浆中可见小胶质细胞浸入

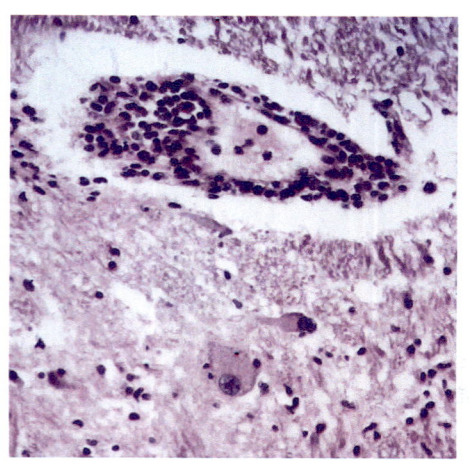

图423　乙脑时淋巴血管套
Epidemic encephalitis B, lymphocytes infiltrating around vessel
血管周围间隙增宽，以淋巴细胞为主的炎细胞围绕血管呈套袖状浸润

图 424 乙脑时胶质细胞结节
Epidemic encephalitis B,
nodule of glial cells
增生的胶质细胞集聚成群，形成胶质细胞结节

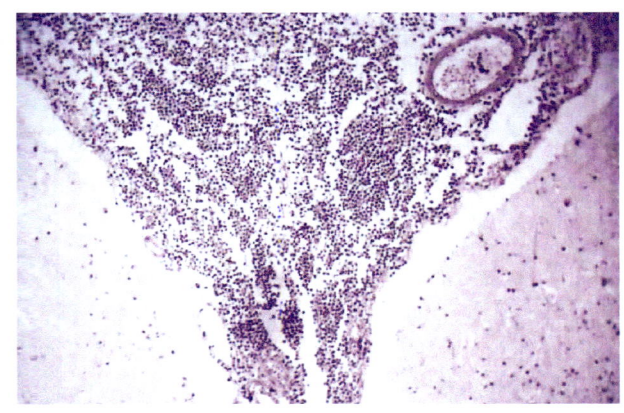

图 425 流行性脑脊髓膜炎
Epidemic cerebrospinal meningitis
镜下见蛛网膜下腔血管扩张充血，大量中性粒细胞浸润

图 426 尖锐湿疣
Condyloma acuminatum
表皮角质层轻度增生，几乎全部为角化不全细胞，棘层肥厚，有乳头状瘤样增生

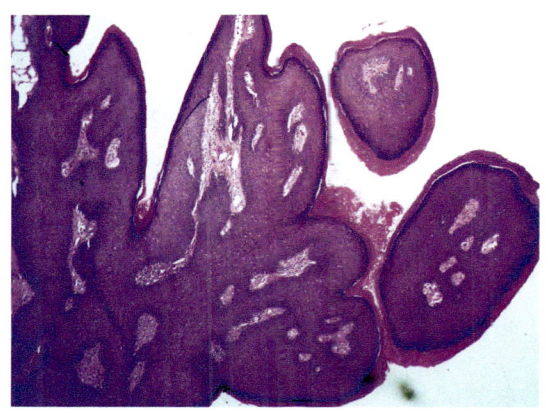

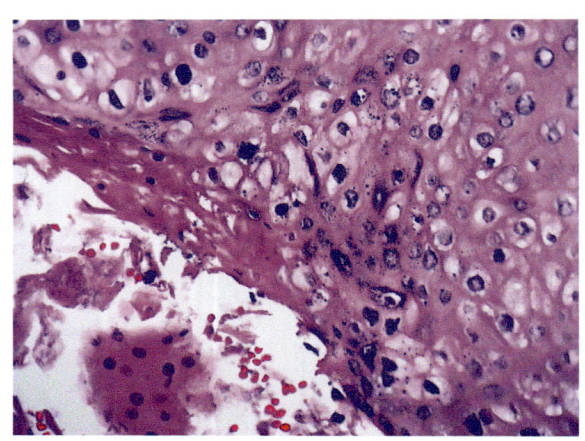

图 427　尖锐湿疣
Condyloma acuminatum
表皮浅层可见凹空细胞，凹空细胞体积较大，胞质空泡状，
核大居中，圆形或椭圆形，染色深

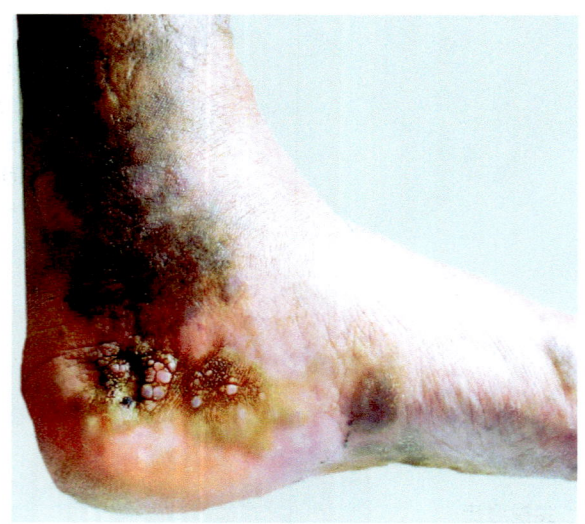

图 428　卡波西肉瘤
Kaposi's sarcoma
AIDS 常继发此肿瘤。可广泛累及皮肤等组织，以下肢最多
见。肉眼观肿瘤呈暗蓝色结节